INTRODUCTION TO RADIOTHERAPY

INTRODUCTION TO RADIOTHERAPY

SAMEER A. RAFLA-Demetrious, M.D., Ph.D.
Director of Department of Radiation Therapy,
Methodist Hospital, Brooklyn, New York

MARVIN ROTMAN, M.D.
Director of Division of Radiotherapy, Department of Radiology,
New York Medical College, New York, New York

with 81 *illustrations*

SAINT LOUIS
THE C. V. MOSBY COMPANY
1974

Copyright © 1974 by The C. V. Mosby Company

All rights reserved. No part of this book may be reproduced in any manner without written permission of the publisher.

Printed in the United States of America

Distributed in Great Britain by Henry Kimpton, London

Library of Congress Cataloging in Publication Data

Rafla-Demetrious, Sameer.
    Introduction to radiotherapy.

    1. Radiotherapy. I. Rotman, Marvin, joint author. II. Title. [DNLM: 1. Radiotherapy. WN450 R138i]
RM859.R33   616.9'92'0642   74-12456
ISBN 0-8016-4070-9

VH/VH/VH 9 8 7 6 5 4 3 2 1

To my wife
MARIE JACQUELINE

Sameer Rafla

To the memory of my father
DR. HERMAN Z. ROTMAN

Marvin Rotman

PREFACE

While conducting radiotherapy instruction courses for medical students, technicians, and residents in surgery, gynecology, and oncology, we became acutely aware of a need for a text on this subject. There is a general agreement that the subject matter is replete with pitfalls that can trap the student, especially when physics, radiation biology, and radiation treatment planning is under discussion. Available texts have not relieved the situation, as most of them soon become bogged down in abstract biology, comparative oncology, and detailed physics and mathematics.

Our objectives here are to introduce the discipline of radiotherapy in such a way as to unravel some of the many complexities that surround it and to get the student to appreciate its scope. Radiotherapy is a discipline in itself rather than just another subject for study, and as such its students must understand the basic sciences related to it, such as physics and biology, in addition to its clinical aspects. However, our coverage on any of these subjects is not meant to be comprehensive or totally inclusive. Since the book is meant to introduce the discipline in a practical applied atmosphere, physics is presented as it is used in radiotherapy rather than discussed in classic, abstract fashion. Radiobiology is discussed in a logical sequence, that is, the effects of radiation on the cell, the tissue, the organ, and the whole organism. A chapter on the biological effects of radiation on malignant neoplasms concludes the radiobiology section.

Since our objective is to introduce the discipline of radiotherapy, we sought to limit the discussion of clinical oncology to material related directly to radiotherapy. This proved difficult, but we were guided by some basic criteria: the frequency with which a particular tumor is referred to radiotherapy, the importance of the role of radiotherapy in the management of particular tumors, and the degree or promise of success that treatment by this discipline has achieved.

The chapter introducing neoplasia seeks to present some of the basic principles common to most neoplastic disorders, particularly the malignant ones. The scheme followed is pursued systematically in the subsequent chapters of this section where the following points are discussed: incidence, age and sex prevalence, histological types, spread, pathological complications, clinical staging, pertinent investigations, treatment and its complications, and prognosis. Although most of these aspects are established with regards to the majority of tumors, controversy still surrounds certain disorders. Wherever such a situation exists, we have turned to the prevalent opinion among radiotherapists. We recognize that this may neither be the only approach, nor even accepted widely by other disciplines, but we believe that an introductory text such as this must support the radiotherapy point of view and its reasoning.

We have also dealt with the anatomy of a radiotherapy department and how it works. This is aimed at explaining to physicians the logistics in a radiotherapy department in the hope that they will then be in a better position to comprehend its various components and how they affect their patients. Its benefit to a technician is self-explanatory.

This work is but one attempt among others at making radiotherapy a more comprehensible discipline, for it is only through its appreciation and understanding by related disciplines that radiation therapy will occupy its proper place in medicine.

Sameer Rafla
Marvin Rotman

CONTENTS

Historical review, 1

SECTION ONE RADIOTHERAPY EQUIPMENT AND APPLIED PHYSICS

1. Radiotherapy equipment, beams, and applied physics, 7
2. Dynamics of a radiotherapy department, 27
3. Planning of radiotherapy treatment, 30

SECTION TWO BIOLOGICAL EFFECTS OF RADIATION

4. Effects of radiation on cells, 51
5. Effect of radiation on tissues, 56
6. Effect of radiation on the whole body, 70
7. Effect of radiation on malignant tumors, 74

SECTION THREE CLINICAL RADIATION ONCOLOGY

8. Introduction to neoplasia, 81
9. Air and food passages, 85
10. Breast malignancies, 107
11. Female genital system, 113
12. Male genital system, 123
13. Urinary system, 128
14. Lymphoreticular system, 134

15 Central nervous system, 139

16 Tumors of bone and cartilage, 146

17 Malignant soft-tissue tumors, 151

18 Childhood malignant solid tumors, 154

19 Skin, 158

Glossary, 162

INTRODUCTION TO RADIOTHERAPY

HISTORICAL REVIEW

The lineage of radiotherapy physics can be traced back to the year 1646 when Otto von Guericke constructed the first practical vacuum pump. With the availability of high voltages made possible by the induction coil invented by Sturgeon and Page in 1836, the stage was set for the discovery of x rays. In 1850 Plucker observed a green fluorescence in an apparatus incorporating a high voltage between plates separated by a vacuum, and he probably exposed himself to x rays without being aware of doing so. In 1895 Wilhelm Konrad von Roentgen, professor of physics in Würzburg, Germany, working with a very similar apparatus, observed the same fluorescence but also discovered the x rays that were being generated as well. This outstanding scientist who was honored by titling the new science "roentgenology" was something of a scholastic misfit. He did not complete his high school education and was expelled for improper behavior but finally succeeded in entering the polytechnical school in Zurich and was later accepted for an academic career. His discovery prompted wide interest in the field of medicine. In February 1896, the Journal of the American Medical Association suggested that x rays might have therapeutic possibilities. In 1900 Stenbeck of Sweden used x rays to cure a histologically proved carcinoma of the cheek. By then Roentgen became an eminent scientist and a Nobel Prize laureate.

The history of radium technology after the discovery of radium is closely interwoven with the history of x-ray technology. The French philosopher and mathematician Poincaré in 1895 speculated on the association of x rays with the visible fluorescence noticed in early x-ray tubes (attributable to the lack of a real vacuum), and he suggested that certain minerals that showed a similar fluorescence might be generating x rays as well. This insight proved erroneous but did lead Becquerel in 1896 to the discovery of radioactivity. Two years later in July 1898 Marie and Pierre Curie, working in the same laboratory, discovered polonium and in December of the same year discovered radium.

Radiation erythema was noticed by Becquerel when he received a burn from carrying a tube of radium in his vest pocket, and Pierre Curie deliberately induced a similar reaction in his arm in order to study the radiation effects more closely. In 1901 radium was used for the treatment of discoid lupus in the Hôpital de St. Louis in Paris. In 1903 Alexander Graham Bell saw the potential use of radium in medicine and suggested that the powder be placed in glass tubes and "inserted into the very heart of cancer." Robert Abbe, a New York surgeon, brought radium to America in 1906. He measured the radium dosimetry by applying the radium to his own skin and evaluated the extent of the erythematous reaction. He later published articles on the use of radium in benign uterine hemorrhage. In 1910 interstitial radium needles were used and reports of sterilization of cancer were forthcoming.

Radium's very unusual properties and its power to cure some cancers caused it to be regarded as a panacea for mankind. Ra-

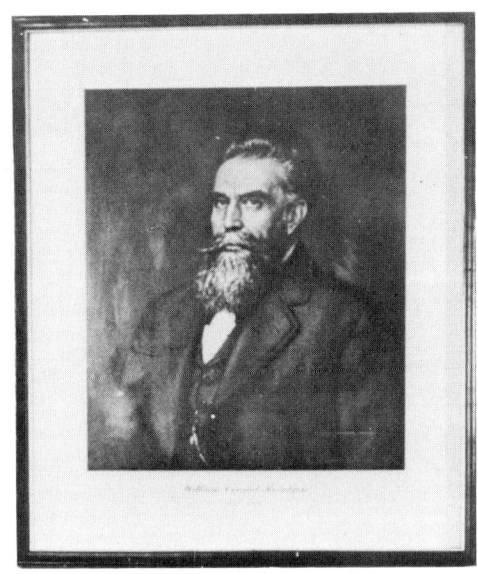

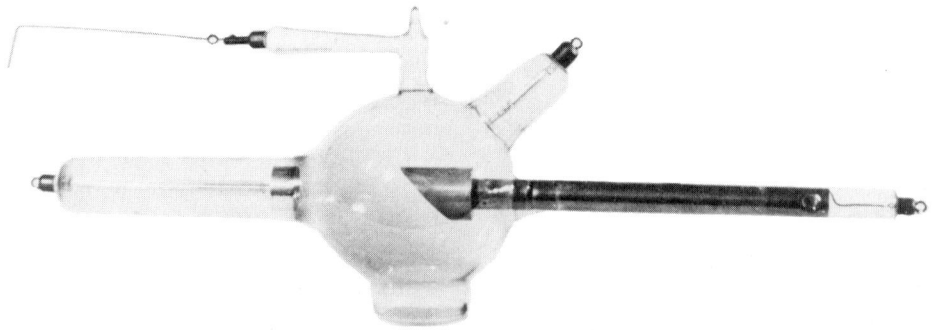

FIG. 1. Portrait of Roentgen and early x-ray tube. This tube was made by Green and Bauer (circa 1900) in Hartford, Connecticut. It has a lead glass bottle (opaque to x rays) and a crown extension (at bottom) for the exit of x rays. The wire (on top) was used as an adjustable sparking device to regulate the kilovoltage. This tube has a tungsten target imbedded in a copper anode. (From the collection of Dr. W. H. Shehadi, Byram, Conn.)

dium was proclaimed a cure for gout and rheumatism and was supposed to possess marvelous rejuvenative powers. One company bottled and sold a preparation called Radithor, which supposedly contained radium dissolved in water and "cured" everything from poison ivy to leukemia. This form of advertising was stopped after several people died from drinking the Radithor. Other companies manufactured radium facial creams, tablets, and suppositories. It was only in the mid-1930s that the American Radium Society resolved that mail-order radium treatment was unethical.

Many believed that radium drew its energy from the atmosphere or from the ether and was called the source of cosmic energy, the sun's heat, and the earth's internal heat. They believed that the myth of the philosopher's stone was founded in radium. Such articles appearing in Harper's magazine included both *Radium the Revealer,* and *Radium the Earth's Internal Heat.* Mention of such philosophic and quasi-scientific thought and enthusiasm lasted through the 1920s and into the early 1930s.

In 1912 Dr. H. H. Janeway was placed in charge of radium therapy at Memorial Hospital in New York. It is believed that he was the first man to advocate radium treatment in the United States as the treatment of choice in cancer of the cervix. His work in this field was significantly responsible for progress during these early years. By 1918 in the United States, Janeway and, in Germany, Friederick, a student of Roentgen and a distinguished radiation physicist, worked out the basic proper dosage for radon seeds (a radium by-product) and used them extensively for all types of cancer. That same year, the first teletherapy radium machine was installed at Memorial Hospital. The foundation of modern radiotherapy had been laid.

The development of radiation physics continued unabated in the twentieth century after having been interrupted by the First World War. In 1932 several important discoveries were made. H. C. Urey discovered heavy hydrogen and J. Chadwick discovered the neutron. In 1932 E. O. Lawrence invented the cyclotron, a revolutionary x-ray machine in which an ion is accelerated in a cyclic fashion by a rather small potential to impart a high final energy. In the following year C. D. Anderson discovered the positron. F. Joliot-Curie and I. Joliot-Curie, the second generation of the Curies, produced artificial radioactivity. It was in honor of the Curie achievements that the Curie was adopted as the unit of artificial radioactive material or isotopes. Roentgen achieved a similar eminence when in 1937 an international dose unit for x-ray or gamma radiation was named after him. The rad, another important unit of radiation dosimetry, was adopted by the Seventh International Congress of Radiology as the unit of absorbed dose of any ionizing radiation.

By the beginning of the Second World War D. W. Kerst finally succeeded in constructing the betatron in 1940. Project Manhattan, which had its foundation in Einstein's early work in 1905, finally produced its fruits in 1945 when the atomic bomb was exploded. This period heralded a review of many of the principles of physics and gave radiation and its effects, especially the damaging ones, a renewed importance. Despite the fact that Madame Curie died of anaplastic anemia in 1934, an affliction that was related to radiation damage it took the tragedies of Hiroshima and Nagasaki to bring this problem to a focus.

There is much to be discovered yet, especially in the field of heavy-particle therapy. The history of radiation and its effects has, by no means, reached its conclusion.

SECTION ONE

RADIOTHERAPY EQUIPMENT AND APPLIED PHYSICS

CHAPTER 1

RADIOTHERAPY EQUIPMENT, BEAMS, AND APPLIED PHYSICS

The methods and tools that a radiotherapist employs to deliver radiation are numerous and protean. They are generally classified as follows:

External radiation
  X-ray beams
    Conventional (superficial and orthovoltage): 60 to 400 kv.
    Supervoltage: 2, 4, 6, 12, and 35 Mev.
  Gamma beams
    Cobalt (^{60}Co)
    Cesium (^{137}Cs)
  Particle beams
    Electron
    Deuteron
    Neutron
    Negative pi-mesons
Interstitial radiation
  Removable sources
    Radium
    Tantalum (^{182}Ta)
    Iridium (^{192}Ir)
    Cesium (^{137}Cs)
    Cobalt (^{60}Co)
    Californium (^{252}Cf)
  Permanent sources
    Iodine (^{125}I)
    Gold (^{198}Au)
    Radon (^{222}Rn)
Intracavitary radiation
  Removable sources
    Radium
    Cesium (^{137}Cs)
    Cobalt (^{60}Co)
  Permanent sources
    Colloidal radioactive gold (^{198}Au)
    Yttrium (^{90}Y)
    Radioactive iodine (^{125}I)
Systemic radiation
  Iodine (^{131}I)
  Phosphorus (^{32}P)
Contact therapy

EXTERNAL RADIATION

By external irradiation we mean **treatment** of the patient by radiation emanating from a source placed externally to his body, usually at a distance. To produce such beams, complicated machinery and equipment are utilized.

Over the last few years, the armamentarium of external irradiation has changed drastically, with the production of beams of variable penetration and characteristics. An ideal radiotherapy department is that which is large enough to possess and utilize the whole radiological spectrum, as this gives the radiotherapist a maximum amount of flexibility by treating any lesion under any condition. Beams used for external irradiation are classified as follows:

X-ray beams
  Conventional
    Superficial: 40 to 120 kv.
    Orthovoltage: 250 to 400 kv.
    Supervoltage: 2, 4, 6, 12, and 35 Mev.
  Gamma-ray beams
    Cobalt-60 beam
    Cesium-137 beam
  Particle beams
    Electrons
    Protons
    Neutrons
    Deuterons

Conventional x-ray beam

The basic x-ray tube is seen in Fig. 1-1 where electrons are "boiled" out or freed from a heated tungsten filament and accelerated to bombard a positively charged tungsten target resulting in x rays. This acceleration is produced by applying a high-voltage. The energy, which is determined directly by the high voltage applied, determines the nature or characteristics of the x rays produced. The main feature that is directly related to the voltage is the ability of the beam to penetrate the tissues; the higher the voltage, the more penetrating is the beam. It may be worthwhile remembering that the fundamental process of the production of x rays when a high-speed electron strikes a tungsten target is a "radiation loss." That is, the electron is attracted to and slowed down by the nucleus of the tungsten atom, resulting in energy loss in the form of heat and radiation (bremsstrahlung, Fig. 1-2). Another important interaction is the collisional loss when the high-speed electron collides and displaces the outer electrons of the atom. These "new" electrons may be ejected from the atom and have enough energy to produce ionization or excitation of other atoms. Fig. 1-2 gives a schematic representation of these interactions. A textbook of physics may be consulted for more details.

The nature of the beam or its quality is directly related to its ability to penetrate

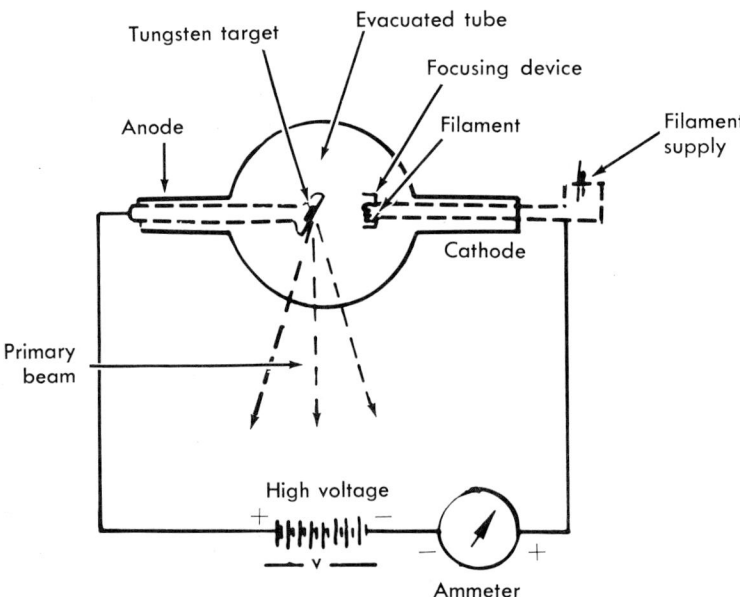

Fig. 1-1. Diagram of the basic structure of an x-ray tube.

matter. The quality is usually expressed in terms of half-value layer (HVL), which is defined as the thickness of some standard material required to reduce the intensity of a beam to one half of its original value. Appropriate materials for the different energy ranges appear in Table 1-1.

Although any x-ray beam is not monoenergetic (see Fig. 1-3), the softer components (or less penetrating rays) are absorbed under heavy filtration and the resultant radiation is nearly monochromatic and of better quality or higher penetration. Such a beam would have a higher half value layer; that is, there is a direct relation between the filter used (and degree of filtration), the quality of the beam (and its penetration), and the HVL. Fig. 1-4 reflects the effect of different filtration on the quality of the beam and its intensity. The choice of the proper filter depends on the voltage applied to the x-ray tube, and the higher the atomic

TABLE 1-1. Materials for different energy ranges

Voltage	Material in which HVL is specified	Filters commonly used
10 to 120 kv.	Aluminum (Al)	Al
120 to 400 kv.	Copper (Cu)	Cu + Al, Tin + Cu + Al
400 kv.+	Copper (Cu)	Tin + Cu + Al

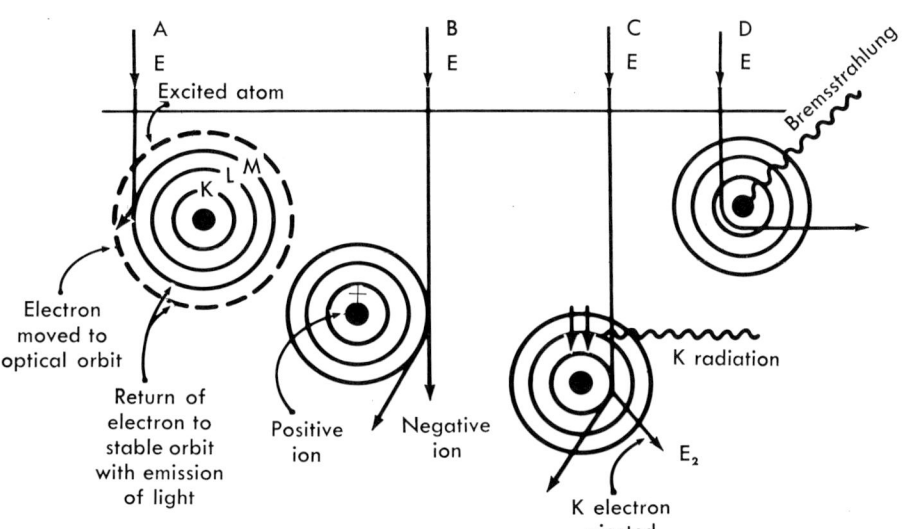

FIG. 1-2. Schematic representation of interactions between the electrons of the beam and atoms in the target in an x-ray tube. E represents the path of an incoming electron along tracks A to D. A, Incoming electron strikes a bound electron and gives it sufficient energy to raise it to a higher energy level but not enough to free it from its atom. This is called excitation. No x rays are produced. B, Incident electron strikes the bound outer electron with sufficient energy to tear it free of its parent atom. This is ionization, and the new electron-deficient atom is called a positive ion. No x rays are produced. C, Incident electron has the energy to remove a more tightly bound electron from the K shell of the atom. When electrons from outer shells fall into the vacancy left in the K shell, they emit characteristic x rays that have discrete energies. D, Incident electron loses energy by interaction with the electric field of the positive nucleus. This energy appears in the form of a continuous spread of x rays with energies up to that of the incident electron. This is bremsstrahlung. (Redrawn from Johns. H. E., and Cunningham, J. R.: The physics of radiology, Springfield, Ill., 1970, Charles C Thomas, Publisher.)

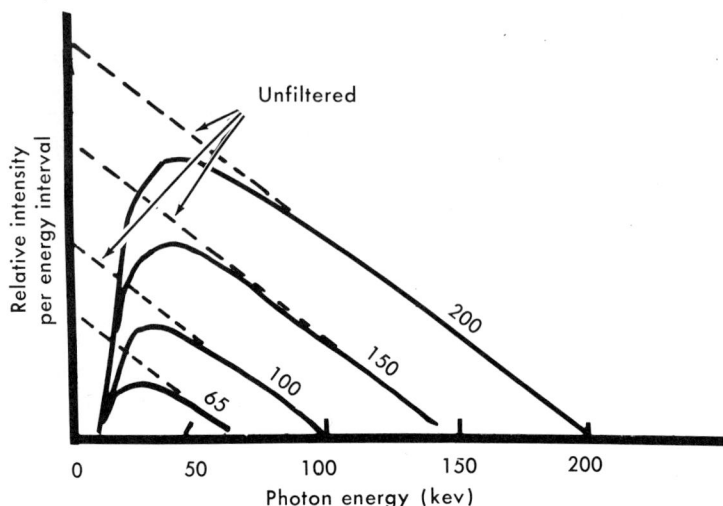

Fig. 1-3. Schematic representation of variation of intensity with energy for electron with different energies bombarding a tungsten target. (Redrawn from Johns, H. E., and Cunningham, J. R.: The physics of radiology, Springfield, Ill., 1970, Charles C Thomas, Publisher.)

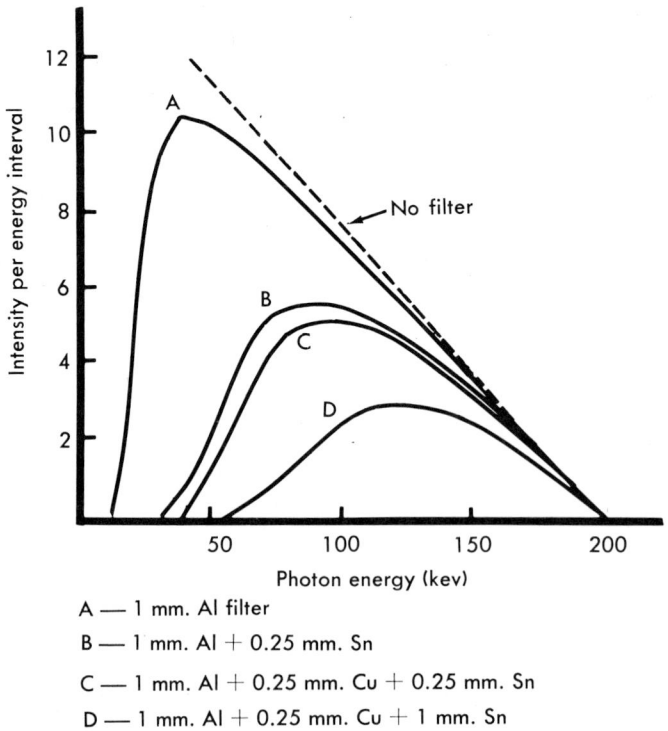

A — 1 mm. Al filter
B — 1 mm. Al + 0.25 mm. Sn
C — 1 mm. Al + 0.25 mm. Cu + 0.25 mm. Sn
D — 1 mm. Al + 0.25 mm. Cu + 1 mm. Sn

Fig. 1-4. Graph showing the spectral distribution of radiation generated by 200 kv. beam under various filtration effects.

number of the filter, the higher its ability to stop radiation. For example, a lead filter (of enough thickness) would effectively stop all radiation from a 200 kv. machine, and consequently it is not useful to be used at this particular energy. Filters shown in Table 1-1 are those conventionally used with the stated energies and are chosen as the optimum filtration to produce the most homogeneous (or as monoenergetic as possible) beam and one of practical intensity.

Since x rays are usually used in treating tumors that are at a depth in tissues, the penetration of beams of various qualities into tissues is very important, and the percentage of the intensity of any given beam at a given depth in tissues as compared to the presumed 100% at the surface (usually termed the percentage depth dose) is of great importance to the radiotherapist.

It is defined in the following equation:

$$\text{Percentage depth dose} = \frac{Dd}{Ds} \times 100$$

Dd is a quantity proportional to the absorbed dose at depth d, and Ds is a quantity proportional to the absorbed dose at the surface. Obviously, a beam emanating from a 400 kv. machine conventionally filtered possesses a higher depth dose than that emanating from a 200 kv.

The conventional beams used in radiation therapy are generally classified as follows:

40 to 60 kv. This "contact" or short-distance beam is so called because the distance from the target (or source of x ray) to the skin is very short and the target is almost in contact with the skin. The beam is of very limited penetration and thus is only suitable to treat skin lesions. Because of the short distance, the dose rate or the amount of radiation the skin receives per unit of time is quite high and so treatment time must be quite short.

60 to 100 kv. This superficial beam has a very limited penetration in the subcutaneous tissues. This beam may be used in the treatment of some deeper penetrating skin lesions. However, since the percentage depth dose of this beam at 1 cm. depth is about 80% and since it diminishes very rapidly in deeper levels, it is unsuitable to treat deeper lesions.

200 to 400 kv. This beam had been for many years the mainstay of radiation therapy machinery. The beam penetration is dependent on filtration, source-to-skin distance, and the size of the field. A representative curve of such a beam is seen in Fig. 1-5.

The disadvantages of all the "conventional" beams are summarized as follows: relatively poor penetration of beam, excessive skin reaction since the maximum dosage is usually at the surface level (for more details see p. 13), and varying absorption in different tissues. The last means increased bone absorption as compared to soft-tissue absorption by a factor of about 6. The reason is that radiation at the conventional voltage is largely absorbed by the photoelectric process. In a unit with a heavily filtered beam of 250 kv., the situation is somewhat better (with less differential) because the mechanism of radiation absorption is split between photoelectric and Compton absorption. This differential is mainly related to the different atomic number of the tissues involved. Photoelectric absorption takes place to a much greater extent in tissues with a high atomic number. Soft tissues have carbon as the prevalent atom, whereas bone has calcium, which has a much higher atomic number than carbon. The clinical implications of this feature are serious when a tumor is treated at a high dose, such as 6000 rads in 6 weeks, since the dose to the bone may reach much higher levels. This may lead to bone necrosis (such as mandible necrosis in the treatment of lesions of the tongue or floor of the mouth) or pathological fractures (such as fracture of the femoral neck after treatment given for cervical or bladder carcinoma). Such complications were so serious that dosage delivered to tumors in these areas using conven-

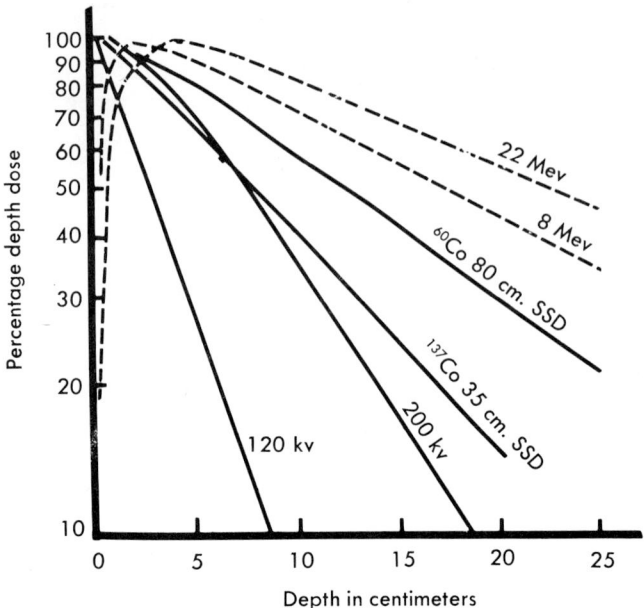

FIG. 1-5. Schematic representation of the penetration of beams of different energies in a tissue-equivalent phantom.

tional beams had to be modified. As a result of higher bone absorption of radiation, any malignant tissue beyond the bone receives a smaller dose because of the shielding or stopping effect of the bone. Because of all these factors, conventional therapy is limited now to skin and relatively superficial lesions.

High-energy (or supervoltage) x-ray beam

The first beam of consequence in this category to be used in radiotherapy was that emanating from a Van de Graaff generator. They usually operate at 2 million volts, achieved by negative electric charges being sprayed over a moving belt to reach a potential of 2 million volts. Particles are accelerated in the tube (by the accelerating electrodes) and hit a water-cooled target to produce x rays. The beam produced is essentially the same as discussed earlier, except that because of the high energy (2 Mev.) it has a high penetration and, as a result of this, is more effective in the treatment of deep tumors. To a lesser extent, it shares with the linear accelerators two more advantages—skin-sparing effect and homogeneous absorption. These advantages will be discussed more fully later.

Linear accelerators are capable of producing beams of 4 to 18 Mev. energies. Beams of higher energy are available. The basic mechanism in a linear accelerator is that of electrons being fed at one end of a tube down which a radiofrequency electromagnetic wave is traveling. The electrons are accelerated to high energy on this wave. These machines were somewhat slow to be widely accepted because of their complexity, but recently, reliable versions have been developed in this country and many departments are being equipped with them.

The main advantages of these high-energy beams are higher penetration, skin sparing, and homogeneous absorption of radiation by different tissues, explained as follows:

Higher penetration of the beam (Fig. 1-5), which may amount to almost double that of the 250 kv. unit, enables the therapist to treat deeper tumors with relative ease. However, such a penetrating beam has the disadvantage of having a relatively high intensity exit beam. The exit beam is that which exits from the body at a point generally located opposite the entry point. This is especially noticeable when a thin part of the body is treated, such as an arm, leg, or neck, where the exit dose may be substantial and may lead to noticeable skin changes.

In the *skin-sparing effect*, the high-energy photons exercise their effect mainly by Compton scattering whereby most of the energy of these photons is acquired by the recoil electrons (see glossary) and the scattered photons have much less energy than the primary ones did. As a result, the buildup of the maximum effect of the rays (or photons) occurs deeper in the tissues, that is, below the level of skin, leading to the sparing of the skin from the full effect of the rays. This skin-sparing effect is very important, as it enables the radiotherapist to treat deep tumors to relatively high doses while the skin absorbs only a fraction. The depth of the buildup depends on the energy of the beam (Fig. 1-5). The higher the energy, the larger the depth; for example, in an 8 Mev. beam it is about 1.8 cm. below the skin surface, and in a 22 Mev. beam it is 3.6 cm. Because of this effect, such a beam is not good to treat skin lesions or deep lesions that have involved the skin (such as fungating breast carcinoma) except if tissue-equivalent material is put in the path of the beam covering the area of involved skin. This would bring up the point of maximum buildup to the level of the skin.

Homogeneous absorption of radiation by different tissues is the last advantage. As explained before, the absorption of radiation energy by a cubic centimeter in bone is several times that of soft tissues in low energy but only fractionally so in high energy, thus the dose to various tissues, whether bone or muscle, will be nearly comparable at the same depth. Moreover, the increased absorption by cells found within the bony structure (such as osteocytes and reticuloendothelial cells) that occurs at low energy is noticeably reduced at this level. Consequently, the complications of radiotherapy caused by excessive irradiation of bone, which were discussed earlier, were considerably reduced with the advent of high-energy x-ray usage. On the other hand, when tissue inhomogeneity exists, such as in the lung, the dose to the tissues beyond the air cavity (aerated lung) increases by a factor that varies up to 30% depending on the amount of air cavity traversed and the position of the tumor and plan of treatment.

Gamma beams

With the development of high-energy devices, such as the Van de Graaff generator or the nuclear reactor, it was possible to produce several "artificial" radioactive isotopes. An isotope is an atom composed of a nucleus with the same number of protons (as the original element) but with a different number of neutrons. Isotopes may be either stable or unstable. Unstable or radioactive isotopes have an imbalance in the number of neutrons and protons that will eventually give rise to the ejection of a particle. The ejection of such a particle is called decay, or disintegration, and the process will continue until a stable isotope is reached. An isotope of cobalt (^{60}Co) and another one of cesium (^{137}Cs) are the most commonly used artificial radioactive (or unstable) isotopes in radiotherapy. The energy released by this decay is called a gamma ray or a photon, which is a bundle of energy that travels at the speed of light (186,000 miles per second).

Cobalt (^{60}Co). Radiotherapy units utilizing ^{60}Co are by far the most common. The radiation emitted has an average energy of about 1.2 Mev. This beam is similar to an x-ray beam of high voltage in many of its characteristics, especially the homogeneity of absorption in tissues. The half-life of ^{60}Co is about 5 years, which means that the ^{60}Co source loses about half its activity after 5 years. For practical purposes, the source may be changed as soon as it has "cooled" to such an extent that the dose rate becomes too slow to be practical. The emanating beam is characterized by having a penumbra (Fig. 1-6), which is the edge of the beam where the radiation intensity falls from 100% to zero. However for practical reasons, the penumbra is the area of the edge of the beam where the dose falls from 50% to zero. The edge from 100% to 50% is considered part of the beam. Some radiotherapy centers consider the penumbra to be from 80% to zero instead of 50% to zero. The size of the penumbra is usually reduced by the use of proper collimators. The larger the size of the source and the source-to-skin distance, the larger is the penumbra. Collimation is carried out by heavy lead screens of about 5 cm. thickness. Ideally, these screens should be put as near the skin as possible to cut the penumbra to a minimal size. However, if this is done, electrons resulting from the bombardment of the lead collimator by the beam will contaminate the beam and, as these are of low energy, would tend to produce excessive skin reaction and spoil the skin-sparing effect of the gamma beam. That is why the collimators should be placed 15 to 20 cm. from the skin surface. The treatment distance, or the source-to-skin distance (SSD), is usually about 80 cm., which would produce a beam comparable to a 2 Mev. x-ray machine at 100 cm. SSD. The source in such a unit varies from 3000 to 9000 curies of cobalt. A smaller source at 80 cm. SSD produces a beam of low intensity necessitating a longer treatment time. This causes difficulty in keeping the patient motionless during therapy, a necessary prerequisite for accurate treatment. A smaller source-to-skin distance would mean such a poor beam penetration because of geometry (inverse square law) and beam divergence that its use in the treatment of deep tumors would be limited.

Cesium units. Cesium-137 isotope is used in these units, the number of which is very limited in the United States. Several important differences between ^{137}Cs and ^{60}Co exist and are summarized as follows:

1. A cesium-137 beam has an average energy of about 600 kv. and is thus

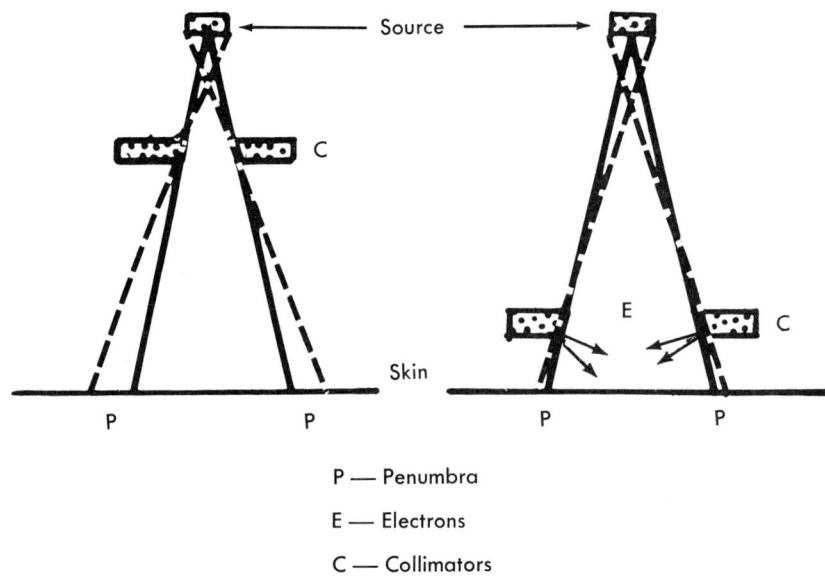

P — Penumbra
E — Electrons
C — Collimators

Fig. 1-6. Schematic representation of a beam penumbra.

less penetrating than that of the cobalt 60. Consequently, less lead is needed around the head (housing of the source) for protection.
2. Because of the difficulty of getting enough radioactivity (that is, low specific activity) in a cesium source, the treatment distance cannot be made more than about 35 cm., and so the penetration of the beam is very similar to that from a well-filtered 250 kv. machine (once again because of geometry).
3. Since the source-to-skin distance is short, the contamination of the beam by electrons (Fig. 1-6) is inevitable.
4. As a result of these factors, the skin-sparing effect of the cesium-137 beam is very limited indeed.

It is understandable then, that these units did not become as popular as was expected when they were first introduced.

Particle beams

Although the x-ray beam is composed of photons, which are bundles of energy, particle beams utilize different particles of the atom, such as electrons (electron beams) or protons or deuterons (proton and neutron).

Electron beams. Electron beams, which consist of electrons, are basically different from x-ray beams, in that the energy of the electrons in the latter are converted into x rays in the x-ray tube (by bombarding a target) and then the resulting photons are converted back into electron motion in the patient, thereby giving rise to the ionizing effect of radiation. In electron beam therapy electrons are deployed directly in the patient body. The most common machine used in electron therapy is the betatron (Fig. 1-7), wherein electrons from a heated tungsten filament are liberated and injected into an evacuated doughnut-shaped por-

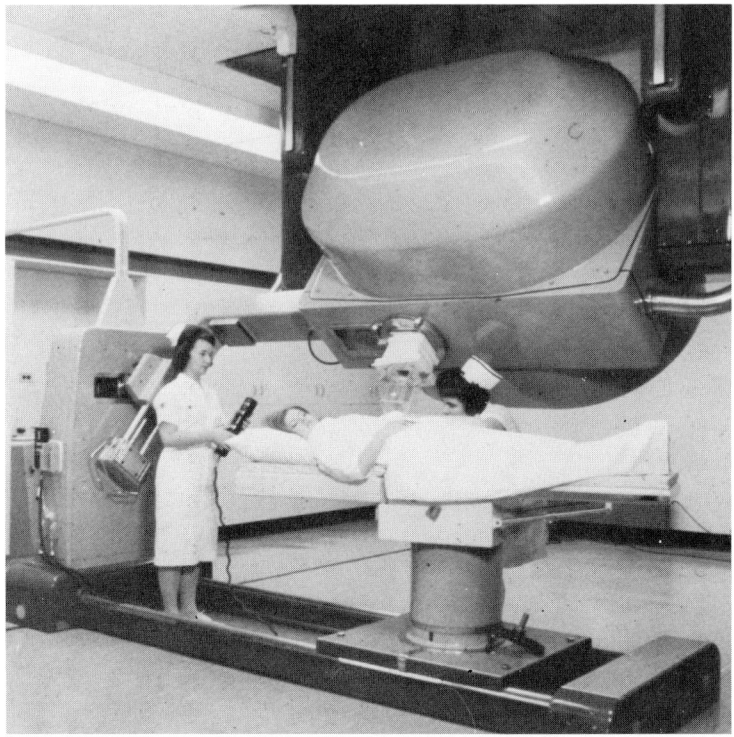

Fig. 1-7. Betatron.

celain envelope. As the electrons travel around in a circle, they are continuously accelerated by a changing magnetic field, which provides a changing flux generating an electric field that gives the electrons a high velocity. If a small tungsten target is bombarded by this electron beam, an x-ray beam is produced with an energy of about 13 to 40 Mev. The electron beam itself may be used after being "peeled off" the accelerating device and emerging through a thin window in the doughnut. The beam may be used at variable energies from 10 to 30 Mev.

The *characteristics* of this beam are summarized as follows:

1. The dose from the electrons is nearly constant to a depth corresponding to the range of these electrons in tissue (Fig. 1-8), after which the dose is rapidly reduced. This range depends largely on the energy applied; for example, 80% depth dose of a 15 Mev. beam is delivered to a depth of about 5 cm. This relation of 3:1 is a rough rule. A beam of 8 Mev. has a penetration of just over 2 cm. in tissues and thus is only suitable for the treatment of superficial lesions. At any energy level, the superficial block of tissues in the passage of the beam receives the effective dose.
2. The maximum buildup is at the skin level, especially at energies below 20 Mev.
3. Bone exercises a shielding effect on the tissues deep to it in the path of an electron beam. In bones there is also an increased absorption of energy relative to that of soft tissues, with the result of heterogeneous dose absorption.

With these characteristics, the use of an electron beam in radiation therapy has been rather limited. For instance, although it is ideal for a fungating breast lesion, it is not so for the treatment of parasternal nodes.

Deuteron beam. A deuteron is a heavy particle (proton and neutron) and like the rest of heavy particle beams is still largely experimental. The beam shows a very attractive feature (Fig. 1-8) in that it affords a small surface dose with the maximum

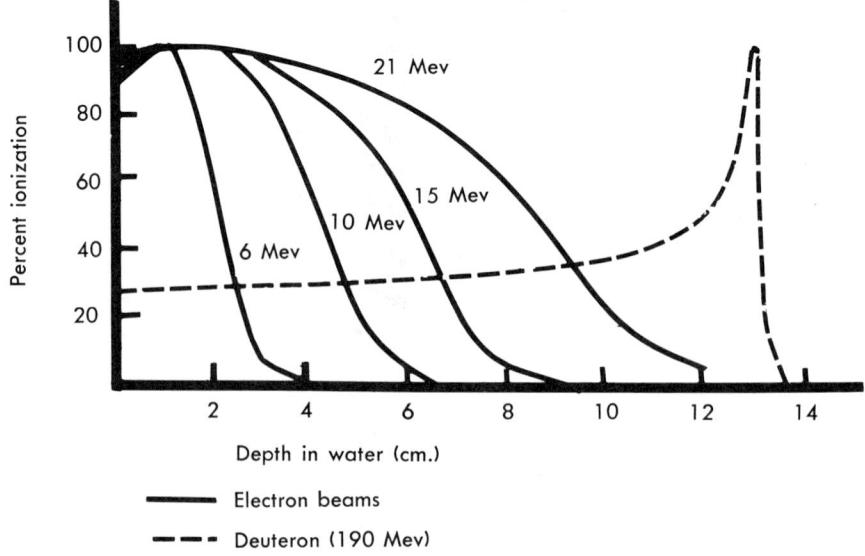

Fig. 1-8. Curves representing penetration of electron beams of different energies.

dose occurring at a depth depending on the energy applied; for example, 190 Mev. deuterons have the maximum buildup at 13 cm. Such a curve is called a Bragg curve and its potential can be appreciated if one can imagine that it is possible to adjust the peak in the curve (Fig. 1-8) to a tumor so that the result would be delivery of a high dose to the tumor and a minimal dose to the tissues in the pathway. Unfortunately, matters are not that simple in practice; the machine necessary to produce such a beam is a synchrocyclotron, which is too large and too expensive to be used routinely in radiotherapy. Moreover, the span of the peak is too narrow to accommodate most tumors.

Neutron beam. Investigation of fast neutron radiation therapy has taken place at a number of medical centers in the past decade. The two major sources of neutrons used include the cyclotron for external beam therapy and californium (^{252}Cf) for interstitial therapy. Neutrons are released from the nuclei of all atoms, except hydrogen, by energetic nuclear collisions caused by the bombardment of beryllium with deuterons. The resultant beam (of released neutrons) shows certain advantages over x rays and gamma rays in radiation therapy. These are a lower oxygen enhancement ratio (OER) (see p. 166), reduced cell recovery from partial damage, and lower differential absorption of the beam in bone as compared to soft tissue. Dose rate and fractionation of this beam may prove ultimately to play a significant role.

Negative pi-meson beam. These particles are negatively charged and interact with nuclei. Pi-meson capture (usually by an oxygen-16 nucleus) involves the meson particle's orbiting around the nucleus while cascading down through the various atomic levels (electron shells) and emitting characteristic x rays just before capture by the nucleus. The x rays produced (mesic x rays) may be used in the future to visualize and adjust the treatment volume.

The beam delivered is broad and shows a favorable (low) oxygen enhancement ratio.

INTERSTITIAL RADIATION

Interstitial radiation is delivered by implanting radioactive sources directly into neoplastic tissues. Examples of such treatment are radium implant for tongue carcinoma, radioactive gold grain implants for carcinoma of the bladder or a tantalum wire implant for a skin carcinoma (such as anal lesions). There are two types of implants—removable and permanent.

Removable implants

Removable implants are those where the radioactive sources are removed from tissues after a certain time during which a specified dose has been delivered. The most common radioactive materials used are radium, tantalum, iridium (^{198}Ir), iodine-125 and cobalt-60 needles.

Radium. Radium (Ra) is a natural element discovered by Marie and Pierre Curie in 1898. It is the sixth member of the uranium series. When radium is isolated from its parent, it disintegrates with a half-life of 1622 years to form radon (see p. 167).

The activity of the radium is mainly (98.8%) through its disintegration to alpha particles of 4.79 Mev. energy, with the rest (1.2%) being through gamma ray activity. However, where radium is used in radiotherapy, it is placed in a container that will absorb all the alpha particles and usually all the beta particles emitted, leaving the gamma rays to produce the biological effect. These gamma rays have a complicated spectrum that can be considered as being equivalent to two lines of energy—0.55 and 1.65 Mev. The mean energy is 1.25 Mev. which is similar to radioactive cobalt. Nevertheless, from the point of view of protection, radium requires thicker barriers than does cobalt because of the higher energy gamma rays. The quantity of radium in a source is always specified in milligrams (mg.) of radium element. The first radium standards were prepared by Madame Curie in the form of chemically pure salts and these standards are stored near Paris. Secondary standards are now available in most national laboratories. Radium sources that are used in implants are in the form of needles; those used for intracavitary applicators are in the form of capsules and are discussed later. Radium needles (Fig. 1-9), usually ensheathed in platinum, come generally in three lengths: short, containing one cell of radium of 1 mg. strength and 1.2 cm. in length; medium, containing two cells of radium of 2 mg. strength and 2.4 cm. in length; and long, containing three cells of radium of 3 mg. strength and 3.6 cm. in length. The radium cell is usually placed in the middle of the needle with both ends being inactive metal. Radium is usually stored under heavy lead protection in lead drawers with each source occupying a single slot to facilitate its rapid and safe handling (Fig. 1-10). When radium is implanted into a tumor, certain geometrical requirements have to be satisfied in order to deliver a homogeneous dose to all areas of the volume implanted. The dose is usually expressed in rads (converted from roentgens), which is calculated according to the system and tables developed by Paterson and Parker in the early 1930s. Implants may take the form of single-plane, two-plane, or volume implants. A typical one-plane implant is shown in Fig. 1-11, where both the inactive needle ends are crossed by perpendicular needles to achieve homogeneity. If such arrangements are not possible, such as in the case of a tongue implant, then calculations should be modified. Double-plane implants are usually advisable when the lesion is thicker than 2 cm. In recent years, lesions large enough to deserve a volume implant are usually treated with external irradiation by use of small field beam–directed plans. After the external irradiation, resultant tumor regression allows the use of a one- or two-plane implant.

A radium implant should be checked radiologically either by film or preferably by an image intensifier while the patient is

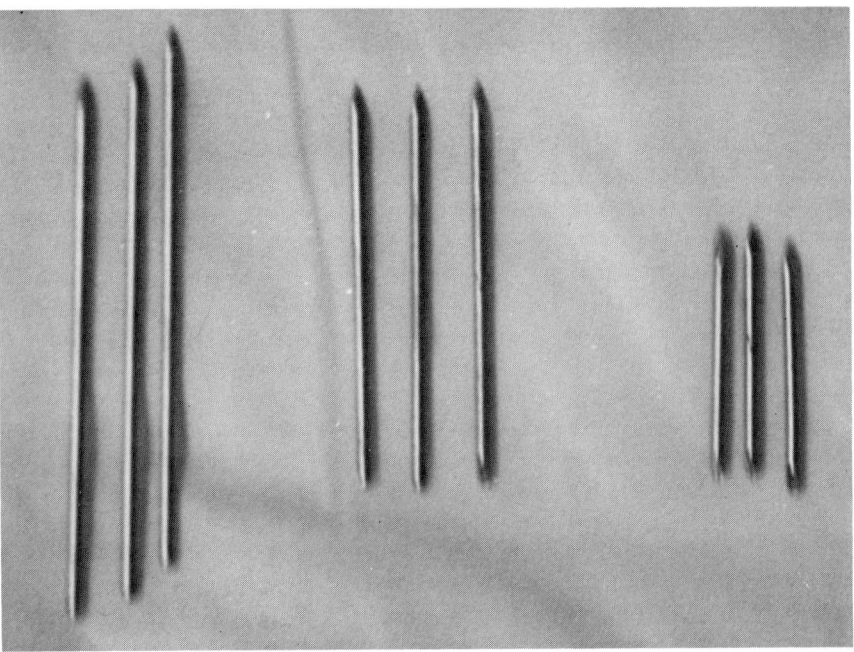

Fig. 1-9. Radium needles.

under anesthesia to ensure that the distribution of the needles is homogeneous and adequate without excessively hot or cold spots. "Hot spot" is a term used to describe a region where there is clustering of needles producing intense radiation compared to the whole implant. A "cold spot" represents the reverse position. X-ray pictures should be obtained and the dose rate is calculated. The length of time of the implant is then decided upon, depending on the dose arrived at. Sometimes, one can mea-

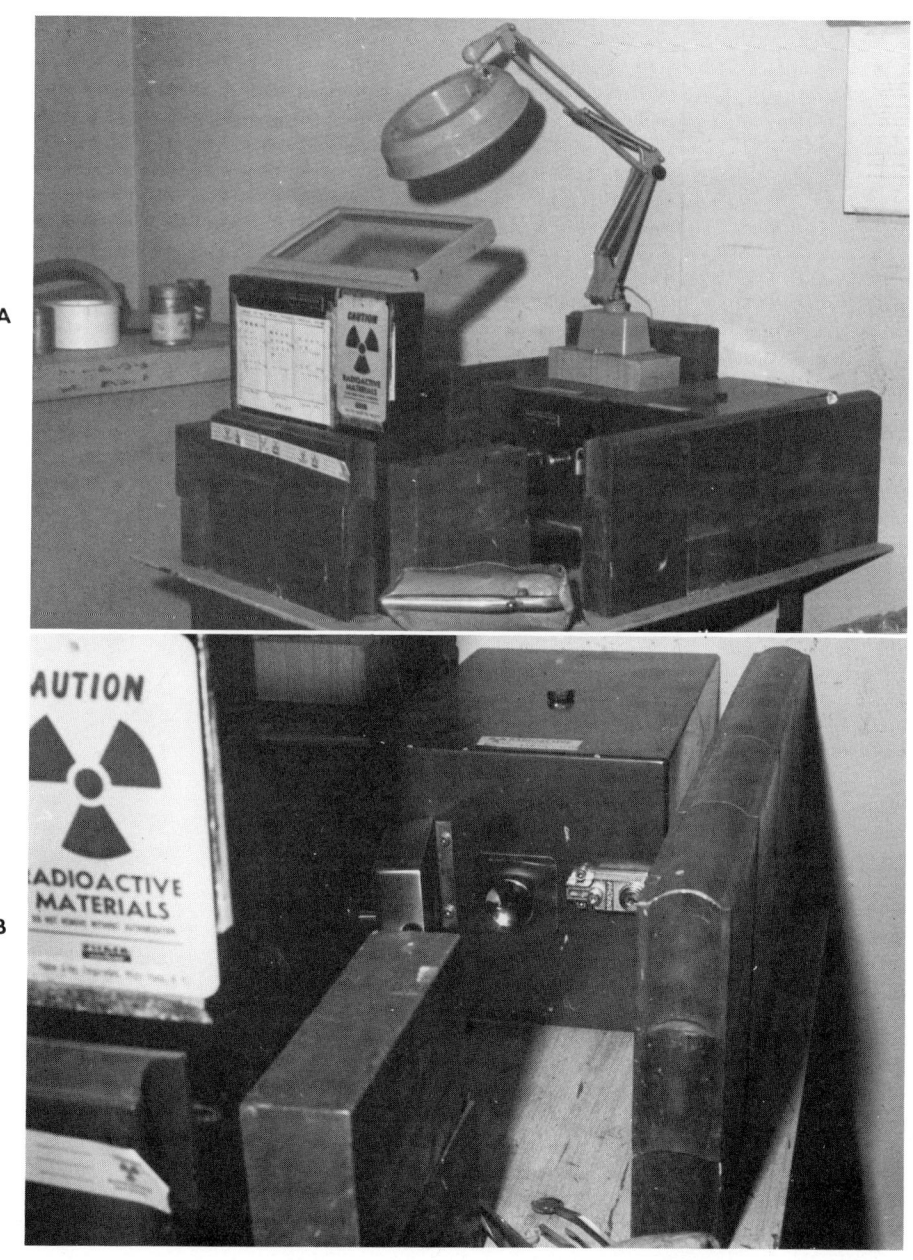

Fig. 1-10. Safe for storage of radium needles and tubes.

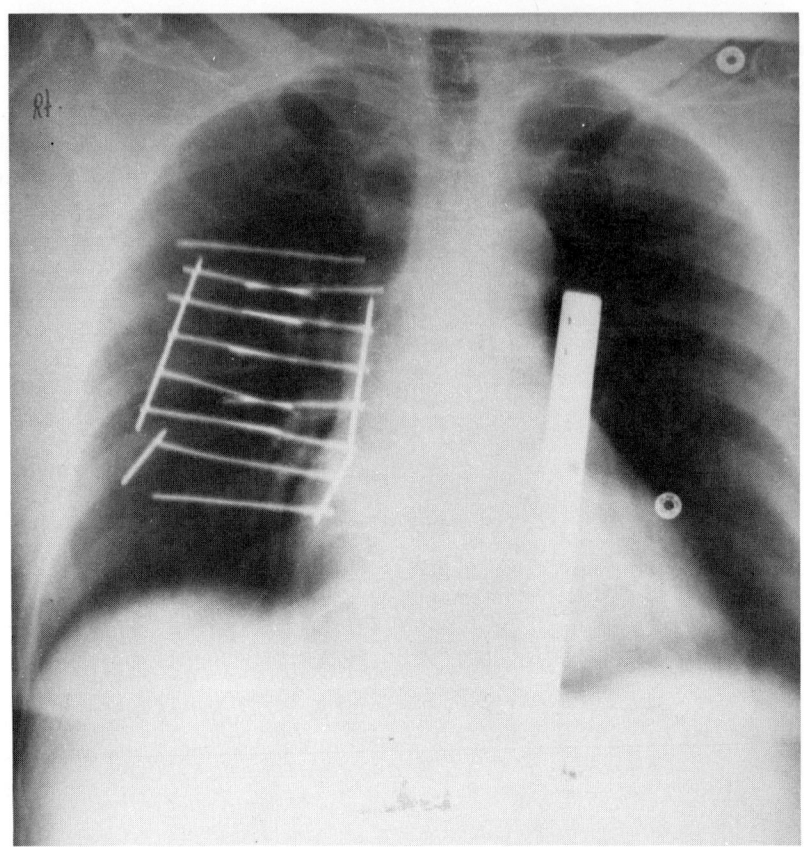

Fig. 1-11. Radium implant in breast.

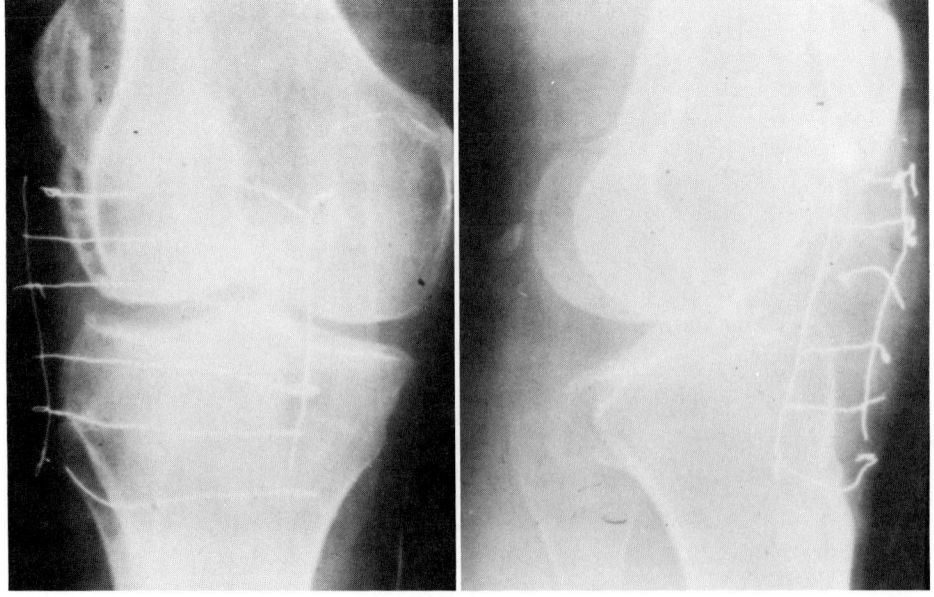

Fig. 1-12. Tantalum wire implant in a lesion in the knee region.

sure the dose given to a neighboring vital structure directly, such as a dose given to the rectum from an implant to a urethral or a vaginal lesion.

Tantalum 182. Tantalum 182 decays with a half-life of 115 days and emits beta particles and a number of gamma rays in the energy range of 0.05 to 1.24 Mev. It is used generally in the form of wires 0.2 mm. in diameter and encased in a platinum sheath. This sheath absorbs the unwanted beta particles, yet it is flexible enough to be molded into a hairpin shape, the form that is in use most commonly in bladder tumors (Fig. 1-12). The technique of the operation designed to treat a bladder tumor by a tantalum wire implant is very simple. The major part of the tumor is usually reamed initially by cautery through a suprapubic cystotomy followed by the insertion of the hairpin tantalum wire by means of a special introducer. The hairpins are tied to an indwelling catheter that is used to withdraw the wires after the prescribed dose is delivered. Tantalum may sometimes be used in implanting subcutaneous or submucous tumors, such as anal carcinoma by the introduction of wires through specially prepared hollow needles employing an afterloading technique.

Iridium 192. For radiotherapy purposes, the element is encased in stainless steel tubes 3 mm. long and mounted in hollow plastic tubes or ribbons. It decays with a half-life of 74.5 days and emits beta particles as well as several lines of gamma rays. The beta particles are screened by the stainless steel and the effective energy of iridium 192 is about 340 kev. Iridium 192 is used in the treatment of some head and neck tumors and is especially valuable in the treatment of the more inaccessible tumors, since the technique allows implantation of the malleable ribbon into irregular shapes.

Permanent implants

The following radioactive materials are used in interstitial implants where the radioactive sources are left permanently in situ to decay completely.

Gold grains (^{198}Au). Gold 198 decays with a half-life of 2.7 days and emits beta particles as well as gamma rays. The beta particles are screened by the case, and the gamma rays are those that are effective with an energy of 410 kev. Each grain measures about 2 mm. in length, and they come packed in special magazines, each carrying 14 grains (Fig. 1-13), which are

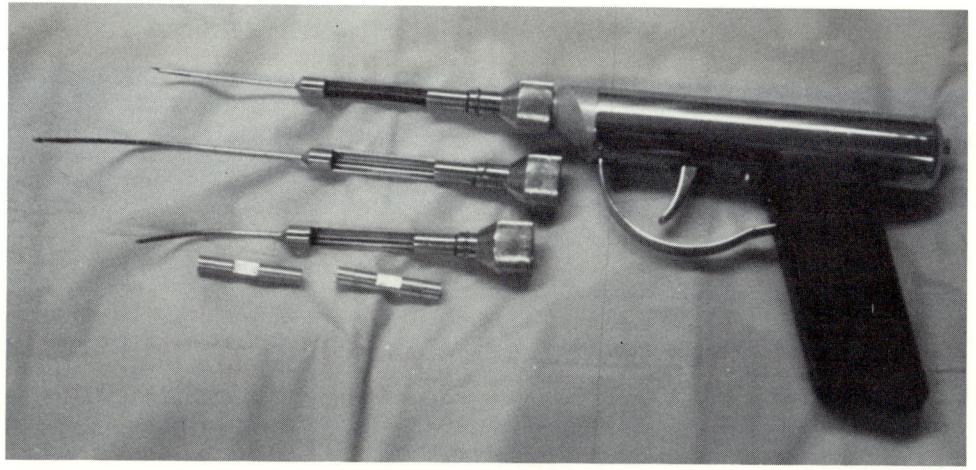

Fig. 1-13. Gold grain gun and magazines.

22 *Radiotherapy equipment and applied physics*

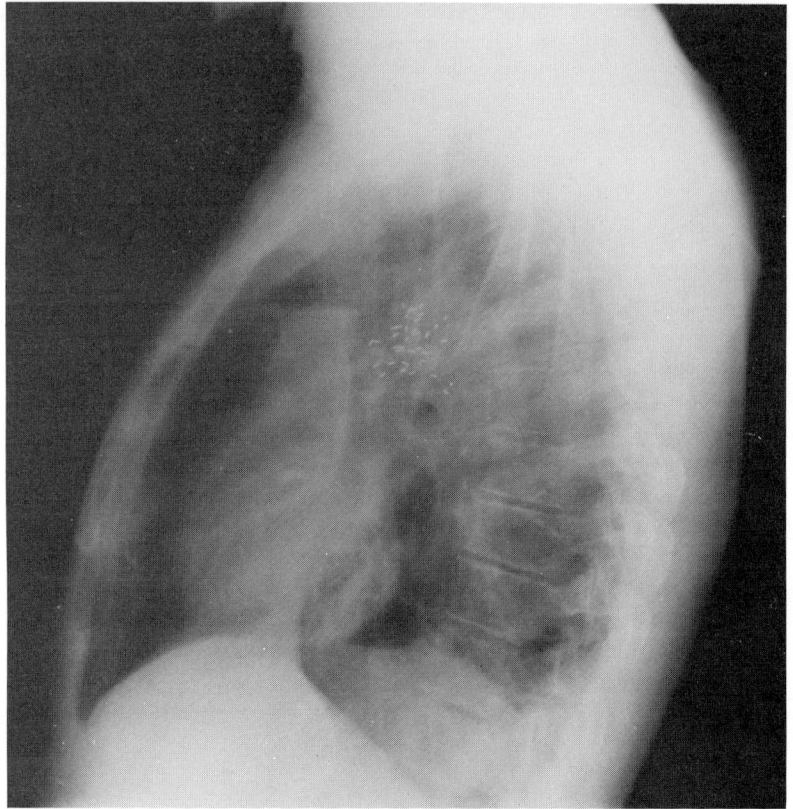

Fig. 1-14. Gold grain implant in a chest lesion.

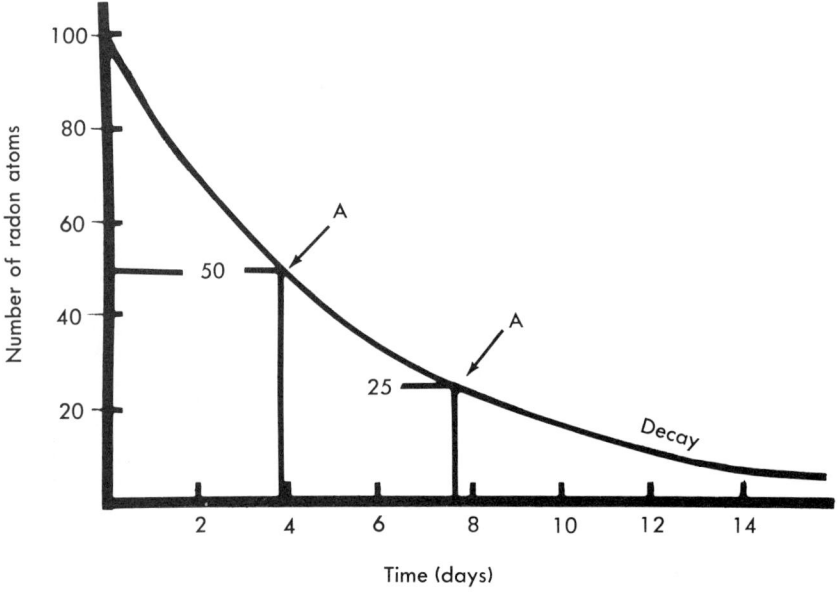

Fig. 1-15. Schematic representation of the decay of radon.

loaded in a special gun, which is then used to shoot the grains individually through the needle. The technique is characterized by its simplicity and is especially useful in the treatment of recurrent or nonresectable tumors (Fig. 1-14). It has the advantage of delivering a very high dose of radiation to a small volume. Consequently the side effects of radiation are very limited even when the technique is used to treat recurrences in a region that was previously heavily irradiated.

Radon seeds. Radon is a very heavy inert gas that belongs to the chemical series of helium, neon, argon and so on. Radon decays rather rapidly (Fig. 1-15) with a half-life of 3.8 days. It is sometimes sealed into hollow gold seeds that are usually implanted, mostly on a permanent basis to treat superficial skin lesions. This technique is very similar to that used in the case of gold grains, except that they are implanted individually.

Permanent implants should be planned beforehand, the volume to be treated studied carefully, and the implant pattern designed and mapped as accurately as possible. Nevertheless, the dose distributions of the resultant implants are usually rather inhomogeneous, and exact calculation of the delivered dose is very difficult if not impossible. That is why the use of permanent implants is usually recommended for palliation rather than for cure. However, hot spots in these implants do not seem to have appreciable, if any, damaging effect. This is probably because they are often very small.

INTRACAVITARY RADIATION

In intracavitary radiation therapy, the sources of radioactive material are introduced in a body cavity. The radioactivity may be *removable*, such as in the treatment of carcinoma of the cervix or of the corpus uteri (rarely in lesions of the esophagus or bladder), or *permanent*, such as in the case of intraperitoneal instillation. Though calculation of the dose is relatively simple in the first case (temporary insertion), the calculation of the dose in the latter is more complicated and usually expressed in quantitative units, that is, millicuries. These factors are elaborated on later in this chapter.

Removable insertions

In removable insertions, the radioactive element used is mainly radium, but cobalt-60 and cesium-137 sources are used on rare occasions.

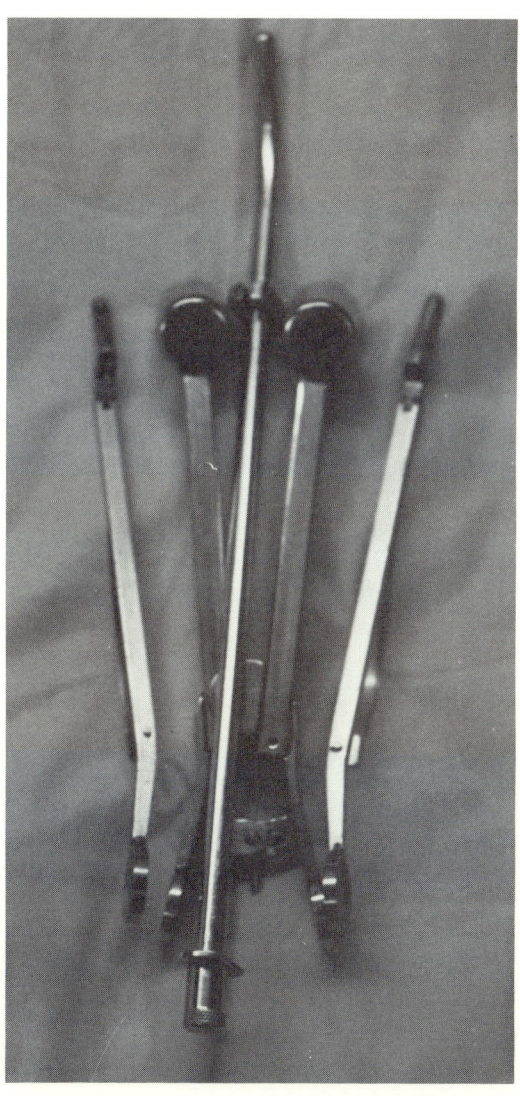

FIG. 1-16. Applicators for insertion of radium into uterus. (Developed by G. Fletcher and H. Suit, M. D. Anderson Hospital.)

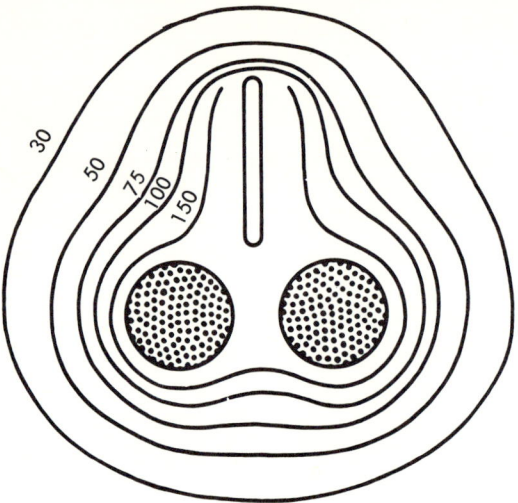

FIG. 1-17. Pear-shaped distribution of isodose curves.

Radium. The element radium in these applications is packed in capsules, each about 1 inch long and of several activities —5, 10, 15, and 20 mg. For the treatment of uterine or cervical carcinomas, the sources are packed into special applicators, which are discussed later. Fig. 1-16 shows the most popular applicators (Fletcher afterloading applicators) in this country. Radium is packed in various combinations according to the type of disease treated and the dose desired. Nevertheless, the general distribution of the intensity of the radiation is shown in Fig. 1-17, which indicates that there is a rapid falloff from the source outwards. The importance and significance of this are discussed in Chapter 11.

Cobalt 60. Cobalt 60 was used in the form of needles for interstitial implants as well as pellets that are used in packing the uterus for the treatment of uterine carcinoma. The half-life of ^{60}Co is about 5 years, and as it decays continuously, its activity has to be corrected periodically and pellets replaced about every 3 years. The main advantage ^{60}Co has over radium is a much reduced cost for the element, but the cost of regular replacements as well as the trouble of continuous calculation has restricted its use.

Cesium 137. Cesium 137 (half-life of about 30 years) has been used in the form of needles or sources for interstitial or intracavitary radiation instead of radium. Its main advantage is cheaper cost. Moreover, the gamma rays from ^{137}Cs (at 662 kev.) are relatively easily stopped by thick lead although they have nearly the same penetrating power as radium gamma rays in the tissue volume usually implanted. This makes protection and handling much easier.

Permanent insertions

Permanent intracavitary insertions are radioactive sterile suspensions instilled into body cavities (such as pleural or peritoneal) when there is evidence of malignant involvement. The three main radioactive elements used are the following:

1. *Colloidal gold* (^{192}Au) with doses of 75 to 100 millicuries (mc.) are injected intrapleurally and about 150 mc. intraperitoneally. The main radioactivity in use here are the beta particles, which have a limited range, with the dose falling to about 15% in 1 mm. thickness of tissues (review p. 21).
2. *Yttrium* (^{90}Y) is claimed to be somewhat superior to gold 198 in view of its higher-energy beta ray.
3. *Radioactive phosphorus* (^{32}P) in the form of 10 to 15 mc. of radioactive chromic phosphate is used in some cases with limited success along the same indications as colloidal gold. ^{32}P is a beta emitter having an average range of 2 mm. in tissue. This characteristic allows its use on an outpatient basis without hospitalization as in the case of the gamma-ray emitters (such as radioactive gold grains).

Intracavitary instillation of radioactive materials is usually indicated in malignant effusions to diminish the rate of recurrence. Theoretically, the radioactive material spreads evenly to produce a uniform dose to the peritoneum or pleura, but this is not always true, since adhesions, which are very common in these cases, lead to localization of the material. Moreover, the malignant tissues in some of these cases may be in the form of thick nodules, which do not receive adequate radiation because of the short penetration of the beta particles (2 mm.).

SYSTEMIC RADIATION

A radioactive isotope injected intravenously may be concentrated in the diseased organ by virtue of selective uptake as in the case of a thyroid lesion and radioactive iodine (iodine is normally metabolized and concentrated in thyroid tissue to form thyroxine and its derivatives). The same phenomenon was noticed in the case of radioactive phosphorus and bone.

The dose delivered by systemic radiation is difficult to measure. It depends on physical as well as biological factors. The physical factors are energy of radiation, rate of radioactive decay, and amount of radioactivity injected. The biological factors are the volume in which the radioactive material is distributed, the concentration of the material, and the rate of biological elimination or excretion.

The dosage aimed at is usually established by clinical experience and expressed in terms of millicuries per kilogram of body weight or microcuries per gram of organ weight (such as thyroid gland in case of ^{131}I given for thyrotoxicosis).

The two isotopes most commonly used in radiotherapy are radioactive iodine (^{131}I) and radioactive phosphorus (^{32}P).

Iodine 131. ^{131}I has a half-life of 8.05 days and disintegrates mainly by emission of beta particles with a mean energy of 0.87 Mev. Nonradioactive iodine is concentrated physiologically by thyroid tissue, and its radioactive isotope (^{131}I) behaves in a similar fashion. Thus an injection of ^{131}I may destroy normal thyroid tissues and inhibit the function of the gland (such as in thyrotoxicosis). The same phenomenon is utilized in the treatment of functioning metastatic thyroid carcinoma. This selective uptake by the thyroid tissue of ^{131}I has also been utilized in testing the function of the thyroid gland (^{131}I uptake tests) or mapping of active thyroid tissue (thyroid scan).

Phosphorus 32. ^{32}P has a half-life of 14.3 days and decays mainly by the emission of beta particles. The mean energy absorbed by the body is 0.69 Mev. ^{32}P is a bone seeker and is particularly concentrated where active bone turnover is taking place, such as in bone metastases (from prostatic carcinoma after androgen priming) or bone marrow lesions (such as multiple myeloma and primary polycythemia). Its ability of increased concentration in some malignant tissues renders it useful in diagnosing certain eye or esophageal malignancies. An excessive dose of ^{32}P is liable to destroy a large amount of active normal bone marrow, which may lead to anemia, leukopenia, and thrombocytopenia.

CONTACT THERAPY

Contact therapy as a modality of treatment is used when lesions are superficial (such as lesions in the conjunctiva of the eye) and full protection to the surrounding and deeper tissues is necessary. Beta rays (or particles) that emanate from radium was the beam first used. Since these rays are stopped by the capsule surrounding radium salt (usually platinum), it was necessary to seal the salt in a shallow metal box where the top and sides were made thick enough to produce adequate protection whereas the front surface was made very thin to allow the beta rays to penetrate. These applicators are called RaD + E applicators, and they decay with a half-life of 20 years.

Recently, strontium 90 isotope (^{90}Sr) was introduced to replace radium. ^{90}Sr is in equilibrium with ^{90}Y and decays with a half-life of 28 years. Shielding of 0.1 mm. silver absorbs virtually all the 0.54 Mev. beta radiation emitted by the ^{90}Sr and also acts as a protective surface. ^{90}Y emits 2.27 Mev. beta radiation and it is this radiation that is used therapeutically. The construc-

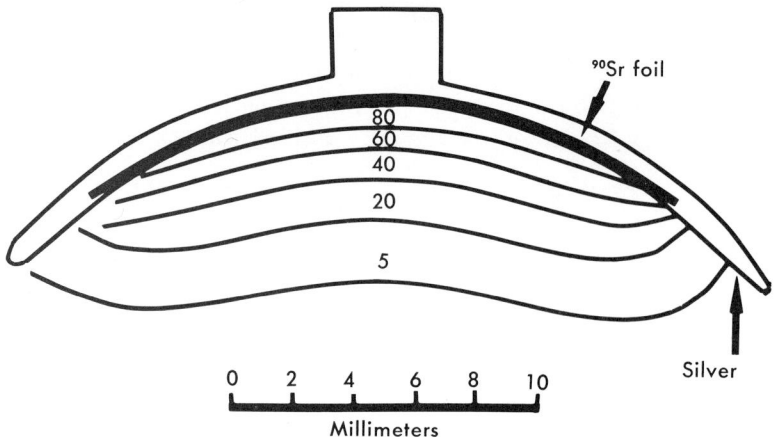

FIG. 1-18. Strontium-90 applicator used for treatment of eye lesions.

tion of the applicator is seen in Fig. 1-18 and the distribution of radiation along various depths (isodose curves) is seen. Such an applicator will deliver the maximum dose (90%) to the conjunctiva or part of the cornea treated with a minimal dose (5%) to the lens (the sensitive structure in the eye).

CHAPTER 2

DYNAMICS OF A RADIOTHERAPY DEPARTMENT

To understand the structure of a radiotherapy department and the dynamics of patient movement, one must appreciate the various functions of the department. Besides training of residents and clinical research, the main function of a radiotherapy department is treating patients. The steps that precede treatment (assessment, examination, and treatment planning) as well as those that follow it (follow-up of patients) are an integral part of its activities.

The basic structure of a radiotherapy department is therefore composed of three interlocking sections—that aimed at patient care, that aimed at training (residents, technicians, and so forth), and that aimed at clinical research. Our discussion here will deal largely with that aimed at patient care. Traditionally, three areas are necessary to carry this function adequately—the clinic area, the treatment area, and the physics area. The functions of each are summarized in Table 2-1.

The type of personnel necessary to man these three areas differs, to a certain extent, with the radiotherapist playing a common role in all of them. The clinic area is usually manned by nursing personnel. Although radiotherapy technicians have manned this area successfully in certain duties, experience shows that nursing knowledge and background is necessary both to facilitate the radiotherapist's job (with their knowledge of various examination techniques, instruments, and so forth) and to ease the patient smoothly in a department unique by its large machines, complicated-looking gadgets, and unfamiliar language. After all, patients are generally used to deal with nurses in all other medical specialties. Whether patients are seen in joint clinics or by one doctor, it is advisable that they should relate very strongly to their radiotherapist during the treatment period, as he alone knows the treatment that will be given, its expectations, and its complication. During the period of treatment the radiotherapist should be the primary physician of the patient. Such a position is identical to that of a surgeon or a gynecologist in similar situations.

The treatment area is manned by radiotherapy technicians as well as radiotherapists. A physicist or a physics technician is

TABLE 2-1. Function of various patient care facilities

Clinic function
  See and assess new patients
    Joint clinics
    Individually
  See patients on treatment regularly
  See patients in follow-up
    Joint clinics
    Individually
    By letter
Treatment area function
  Treat patients
  Make sure that patients treated are seen regularly by physicians
  Transfer to physician their notes about patient, disease, and plan of treatment
Physics and treatment planning function
  With radiotherapist
    See patient to be treated
    Plan treatment
    Apply plan
    Check plan
    Physics activity

---

usually necessary when sophisticated (such as accelerator or betatron) or newly introduced machinery is in use. It is always advisable to have a nurse in this area, especially when very ill patients are under treatment. This is especially indicated in cases of patients who are under oxygen inhalation, with tracheostomies or in any distress. However, it may not always be possible to employ a nurse, especially in smaller hospitals. Thus a radiotherapy technician should be well versed in emergency nursing measures and general nursing procedures. Of course, an impeccable knowledge of the techniques used and complications of treatment is as important, if not more so, as knowing the knobs and buttons of the unit used. A knowledge of practical psychology as well as a humane attitude toward patients is, we believe, still the most important requirement of a successful radiotherapy technician.

The third area, physics and treatment planning, is manned by physicists and physics technicians, in addition to radiotherapists. In a large hospital or where sophisticated machinery (such as simulators) are in use, an x-ray technician who is well trained in radiodiagnosis as well as radiotherapy is necessary. Such a technician is priceless, if one is to make full and proper use of a simulator.

Secretarial personnel are vital for the smooth function of a modern radiotherapy department. Clearly typed, concise, up-to-date, and properly filed charts are no longer a luxury. Special training is important if a secretary is to perform her job adequately. Complete understanding of the functions of a radiotherapy department as well as the structure of its various components is necessary. Intimate knowledge of other departments of the hospital, with which radiotherapy is intimately related, such as surgery, medical oncology, pathology, diagnostic radiology, and social services, is a great asset. Training in tumor registry and the importance of its various aspects is an important requirement.

The dynamics of the movement in a radiotherapy department varies from one center to the other, depending on work load, philosophy and techniques of treatment, and the degree of development of the particular department. Nevertheless, it is advisable that patients are seen primarily and at regular intervals (during treatment) in the clinic area. This does not obviate daily observation and frequent examination during treatment, which may be carried out either in special examination rooms in the treatment area or in the clinic area. The patient usually moves after the primary examination and assessment to the treatment planning area and then to the treatment area. Preferably, definitive treatment should not be instituted until the plan of treatment is finalized and checked satisfactorily. This pattern does not usually apply to every patient and may be modified according to the needs of the patient.

A cardinal fact to remember: Radiotherapy is a palliative measure in at least half the patients accepted for treatment. Palliation is aimed at relieving suffering. Suffering may be physical as well as mental and often both. It is the responsibility and duty of all those involved in radiotherapy to deal with every patient just as he is, a human being in a dilemma who needs help. If the shortcomings of our discipline and facilities are such that we can only cure less than half of our patients, let us at least try to extend a humanitarian hand to all of them.

CHAPTER 3

PLANNING OF RADIOTHERAPY TREATMENT

The radiotherapist, once having made the decision to treat a patient, must now proceed to planning his course of treatment. This step is so vital to radiotherapy that special sophisticated equipment, such as simulators and contouring devices have been developed to help make it more accurate. Planning of radiation therapy consists of the following three essential steps:
1. Localizing the lesion or the volume to be treated
2. Formulating the details of treatment, that is, choice of machine, field to be used, the arrangement, and finally the dose/time to be aimed at
3. Checking the plan of treatment to ensure its proper applicability

These three steps should ideally be carried out before any treatment is applied.

The planning team consists of a physicist, mold room technician (particularly if any beam-directing devices are envisaged), diagnostic x-ray technician, and a therapy technician, in addition to the radiation therapist. The necessary equipment includes a cast-forming device (and other devices for beam direction, Fig. 3-1), a device to obtain an outline of the section of the body to be treated (such as a pantograph, Fig. 3-2), and a simulator, Fig. 3-3. The physicist should be well equipped and acquainted with isodose curves and dose-checking devices, which may include various dosimeter systems and phantom (see glossary and Fig. 3-4). Recently dosimetry planning has been carried out more efficiently by computer.

Now we will describe briefly the above-mentioned equipment.

MOLD- OR CAST-FORMING MACHINE (Fig. 3-1)

The objective of this machine is to create a cast (of the body section to be treated) made of Perspex. This cast, when worn by the patient, serves to immobilize the part under treatment in the same position every time the patient is treated. For some years, these casts were made of bandages impregnated with plaster of paris applied and molded to the part to be treated (Fig. 3-5). Their great disadvantage is their opacity, which restricts the necessary accurate fit to the important anatomical points, in addition to the fact that one has to mark the patient blindly. Moreover, making such casts of the necessary thinness (to avoid unnecessary pressure) and at the same time of enough rigidity, needs a certain degree of expertise that is not always available. That is why many centers have resorted to the Perspex cast (Fig. 3-5). It is made in three steps—impression taken either by plaster-impregnated bandages or by special paste in the case of small anatomical parts, such as the ear. One makes a statue of plaster of paris by simply filling the impression cast and finally molds the Perspex cast onto the statue in the vacuum mold-forming machine. The cast is then fitted to the part to be treated and fixed to a special platform, which was used when the impression was taken. The major disadvantages of this Perspex cast is that it is time consuming, with a total of about 90 minutes for the three steps, performed usually in a span of 2 days. The cost of the whole procedure is modest, and it can be perfected in a relatively short time. The resultant cast is transparent, and so it permits a clear vision of the various anatomical landmarks and renders the necessary markings very simple. Very few patients dislike its use (in contrast to the plaster cast), and almost all of them welcome it, since it spares them the otherwise necessary presence of skin marks.

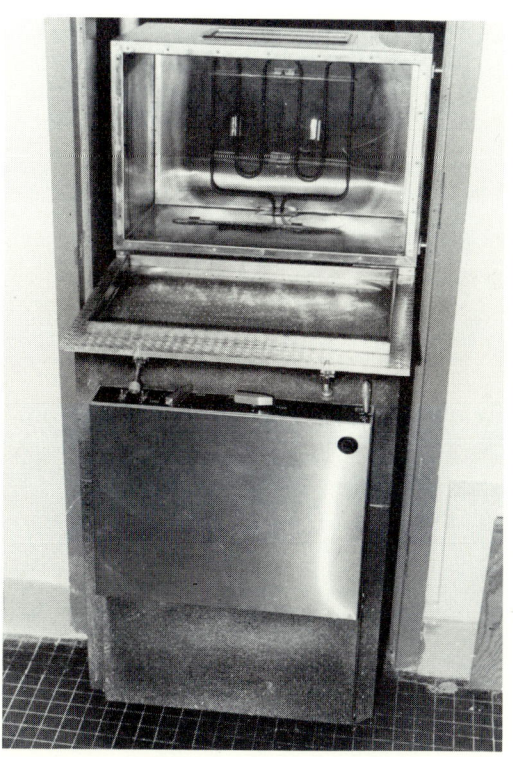

FIG. 3-1. Cast-formulating machine in the last stage of formulating the Perspex case on the plaster of paris statue.

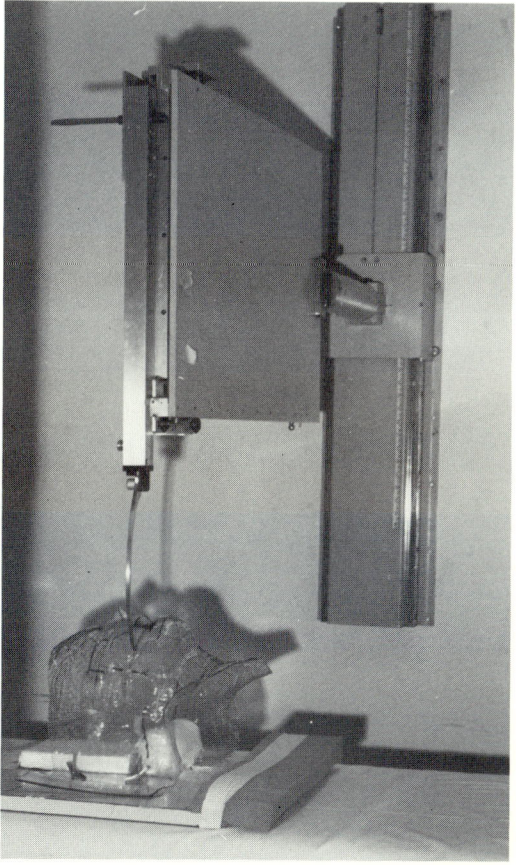

FIG. 3-2. Pantograph, a device used to obtain body outline.

DEVICES TO OBTAIN THE OUTLINE OF THE BODY

Many devices have been used toward the objective of obtaining a body outline. Some of them are strips of lead rubber, solder wire, a series of pins (Fig. 3-6), and the pantograph. This machine (Fig. 3-2) is perhaps the most recent gadget. It has the advantage of plotting the outline of the body at any desired angle that is required to be used in the subsequent planning of the treatment fields (or portals of entry of the treatment beam). It can also mark on the body (or on the cast), as well as on the outline, corresponding points that are used as landmarks during the various steps of

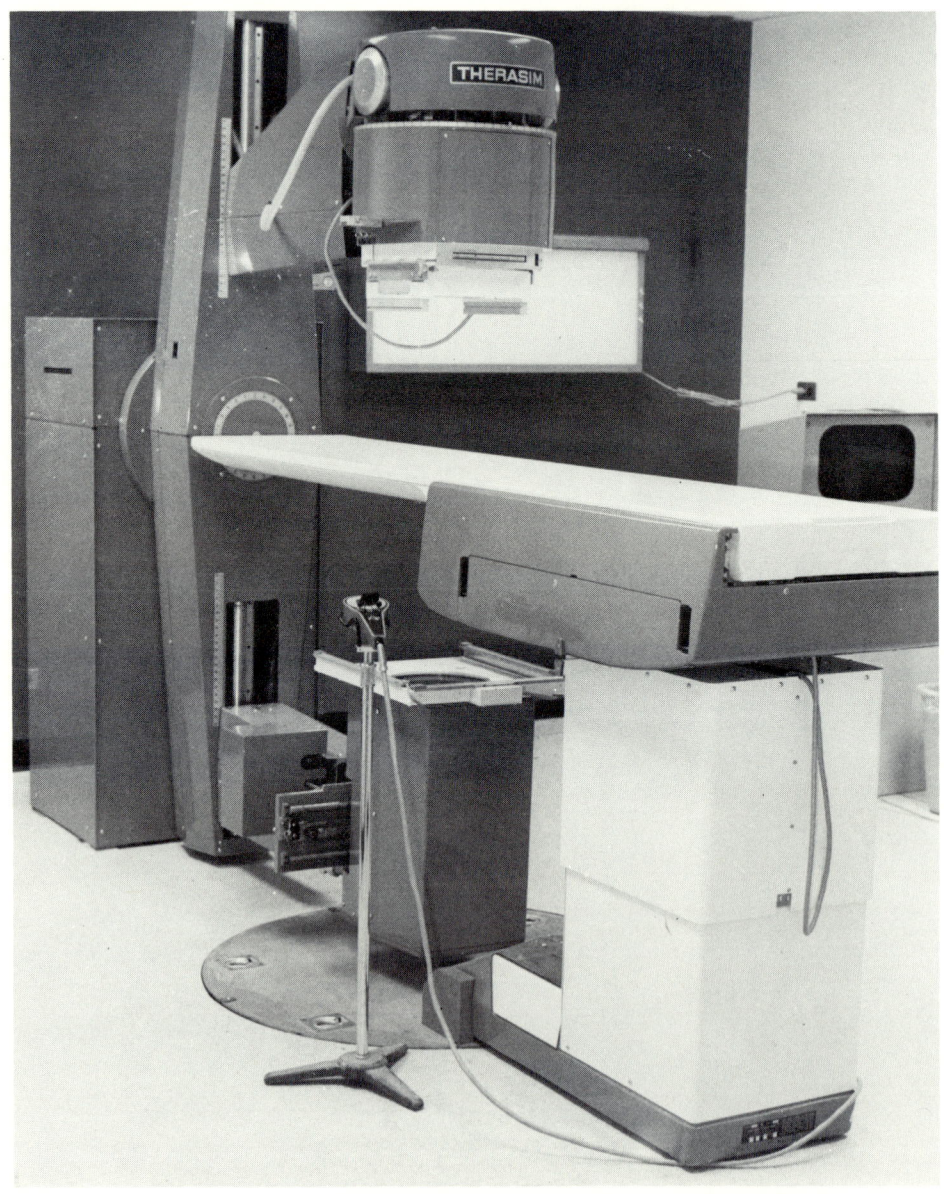

Fig. 3-3. Simulator.

Planning of radiotherapy treatment 33

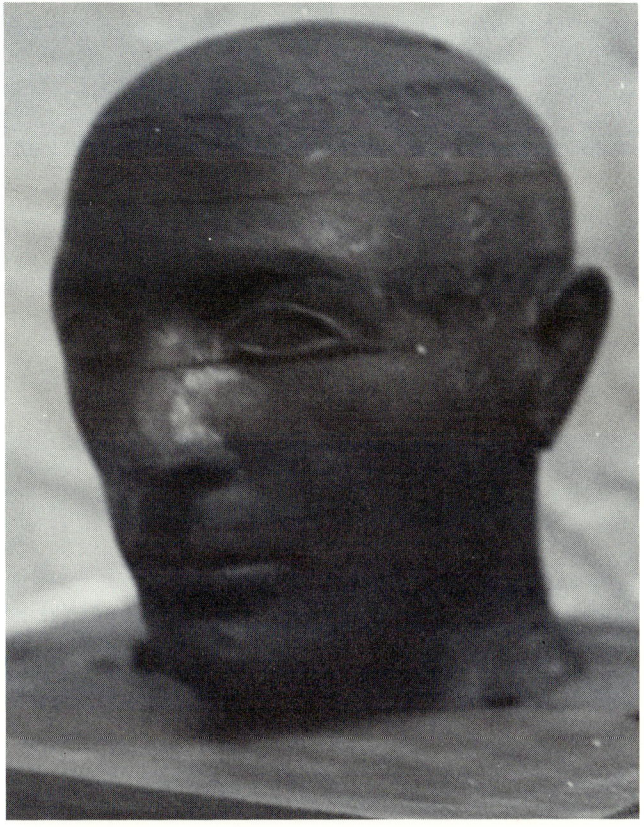

FIG. 3-4. Phantom simulating the human body in absorption of x rays.

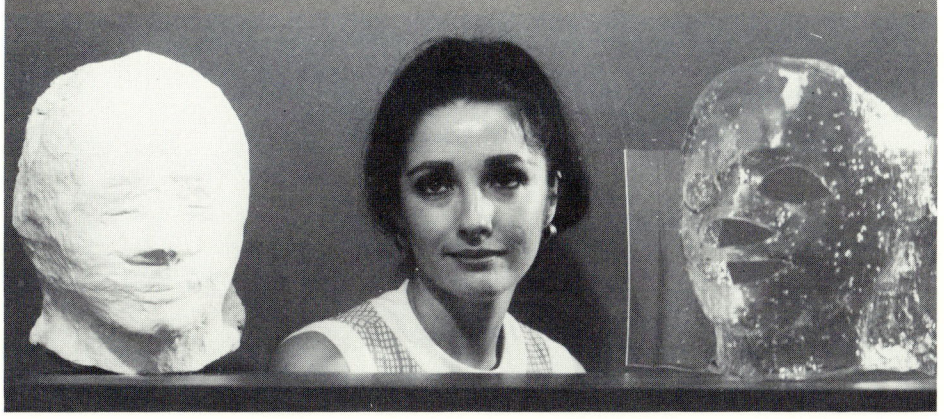

FIG. 3-5. Statue, patient, and Perspex cast.

34 Radiotherapy equipment and applied physics

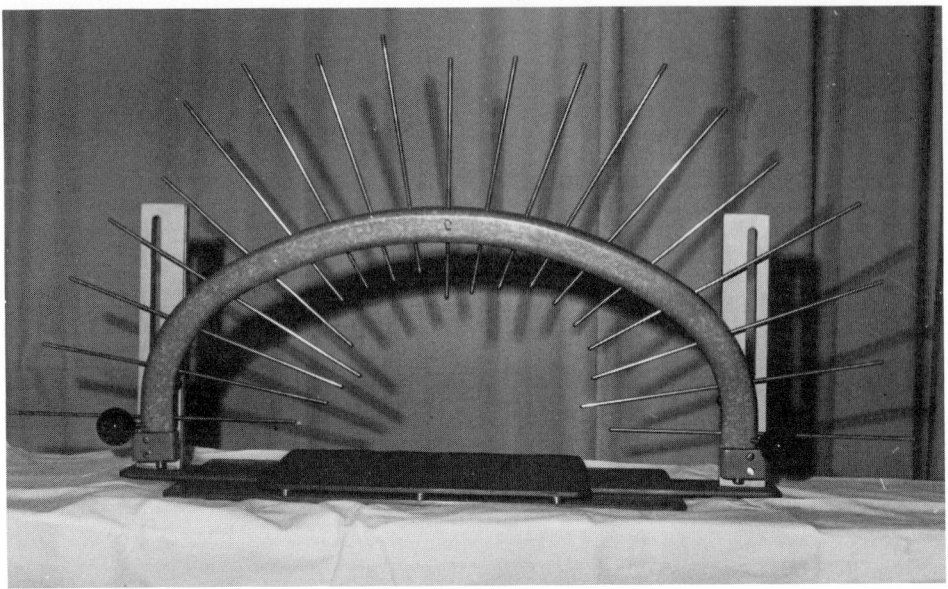

Fig. 3-6. Device used to take outline of body contours by a series of pins.

planning. Since the outline is plotted by remote control, the possibility of distortion (a drawback of using the lead rubber or the pin method) is minimal.

SIMULATORS

Simulators (Fig. 3-3) are basically a skeleton of a radiation therapy unit carrying a diagnostic x-ray head (instead of a therapy beam head) and aimed at reproducing the exact conditions of treatment, such as angle of the beam, field size, and source-to-skin distance. Thus the actual treated volume can be visualized on a television screen (by the aid of an image intensifier) and recorded on an x-ray film. These machines are recently introduced and are not as yet widely used in this country. But since they are very important, their following two functions are discussed in detail.

Delineation of the treatment volume. By the help of the x-ray films and the simulator, the treatment volume can be delineated with marks on the skin or a Perspex cast. The general dimensions of the treated volume should be predetermined by the physician.

Checking the treatment plan. Having formulated an acceptable arrangement of fields on paper (plan of treatment) that is capable of delivering the requisite dose to the indicated treatment volume with minimal damage to surrounding normal structures, the radiotherapist marks these fields on the skin or the cast. These portals of entry are then checked under the simulator by use of both the image intensifier and x rays to ensure that the paper arrangements are accurate and that the treatment volume is in fact included adequately in the area of maximum dose.

ISODOSE CURVES

Isodose curves represent the intensity of the beam at different tissue depths along a single plane (Fig. 3-7). This intensity is measured in a medium (or phantom) that has the same number of electrons per gram as do the tissues, that is, with the same density, and that is capable of absorbing and scattering x rays (or any other beam

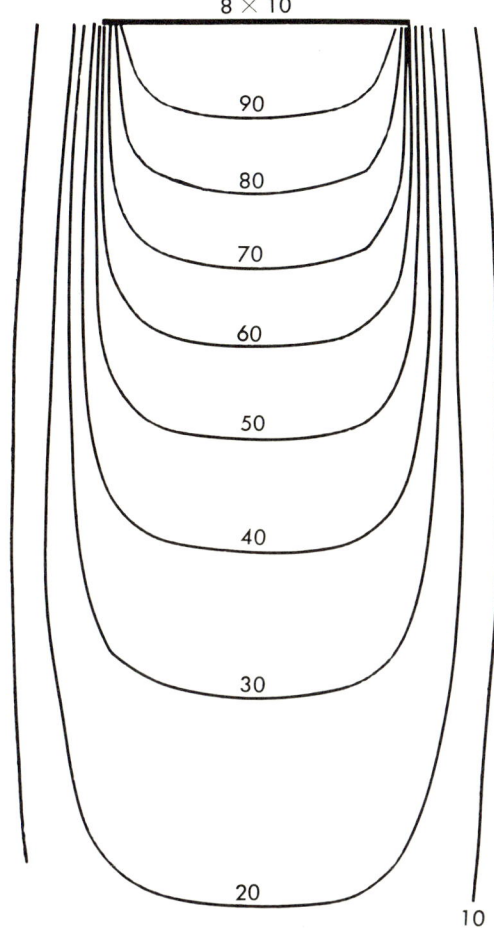

Fig. 3-7. Isodose curve of a ^{60}Co beam with an 8 × 10 cm. field.

in question) like the tissue. Generally, the phantom in common use is water, which absorbs the x ray in almost the same way as tissue does. More recently, a plastic material called Mix D, which simulates water (and soft tissues), has been described. If such a material is placed around a bony skeleton, then a phantom that simulates the body with its bones more accurately than water alone can be built. The latter phantom has been developed commercially (Fig. 3-4) and devices can be inserted at various levels to measure the doses of radiation delivered. However, for practical purposes the method of isodose curves

Planning of radiotherapy treatment

measured in water is the one in common use. Note that they generally have a curved appearance, and as each line is the locus of points that have received the same dose of radiation, then it follows that the dose along the axis beam is somewhat higher than at the edges, because there is more *filtration* for the peripheral part of the beam in addition to less *scatter*. Fig. 3-7 shows that the isodose curves reduce from above downward as the distance from the radiation source increases. One would expect that a line representing the same density, such as a 50% line, is deeper in a 4 Mev. beam than in a 250 kv. beam because of the sixteenfold increase in energy. The dose at any depth in the medium is the *depth dose* at that depth. The isodose curve is a line joining the same depth dose in the medium. The depth dose itself is expressed as a percentage of the maximum dose from a beam wherever it lies. The maximum dose may be at the skin surface in a 200 kv. beam or below the surface, 0.5 cm. in a ^{60}Co beam or 4 cm. in a 22 Mev. beam. The explanation of the cause of this phenomenon has been given earlier. Factors that may affect the isodose curves and depth doses are the following.

Quality of beam

The quality of the beam or its energy determines its penetrating power. Thus the higher the energy, the more penetrating is the beam. This is the most important single factor that affects an isodose curve. Fig. 1-5 illustrates this factor clearly.

Source-to-skin distance (SSD)

An x-ray beam behaves in a way akin to that of a light beam in its relation to the inverse square law, as shown in Fig. 3-8. The dose of radiation (or light) at point A_2 is equal to

$$\frac{A_1}{A_2} \times 100 = \left(\frac{F_1}{F_1 + d}\right)^2 \times 100$$

A_1 is the area at level 1; A_2 is the area at level 2; F_1 is the distance between source

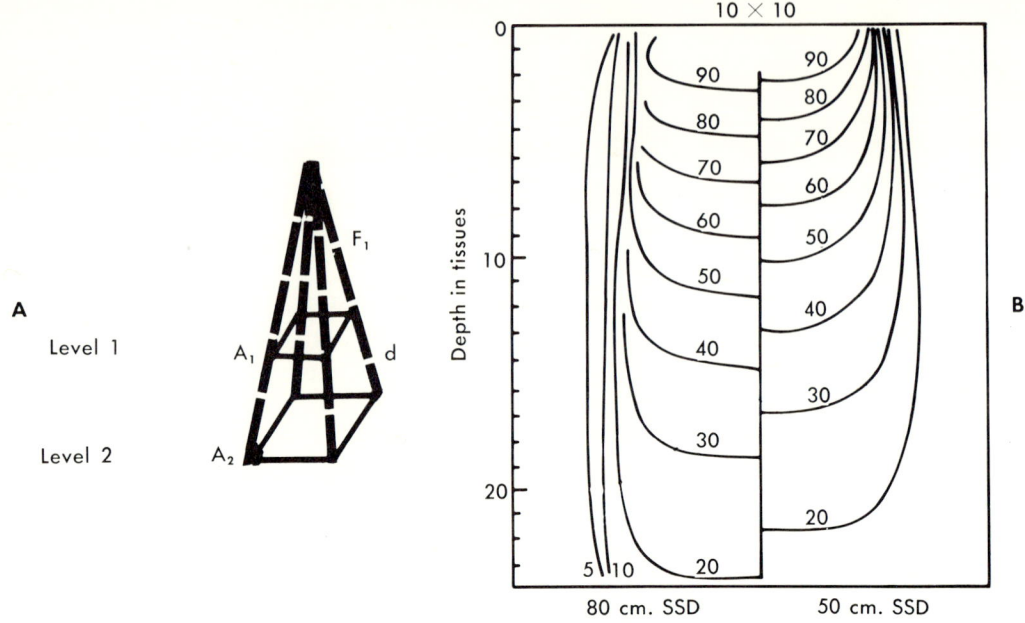

Fig. 3-8. A, Beam spread. F_1, Distance from source to level 1 (A_1). d, Distance from level 1 to level 2 (A_2). **B,** Diagram illustrating the dependence of the percentage depth dose on the source-to-skin distance. (Redrawn from Johns, H. E., and Cunningham, J. R.: The physics of radiology, Springfield, Ill., 1970, Charles C Thomas, Publisher.)

and level 1; and d is the distance between level 1 and level 2. Imagine that level 1 represents the skin and level 2 represents a level in a medium at a depth d, then the dose at depth d is represented by the above equation in addition to the attenuation added to the x-ray beam by the medium. From this equation, it is easy to understand that the larger the distance F_1 is, the less is the effect of d; so, if F_1 is 35 cm. (as the source-to-skin distance in cesium units), then the dose at a depth of 10 cm. without tissue attenuation is about 59%, whereas if F_1 is 80 cm. (as in some cobalt units), the dose at the same depth without medium attenuation is 77%. Thus it is clear that the longer the source-to-skin distance, the better is the depth dose, but the less is the *dose rate* (see glossary) and an optimal medium has to be found. This usually depends on the unit and the available dose rate. A long source-to-skin distance may become feasible; for example, in a cobalt unit with a 5000-curie source, 80 cm. SSD is feasible, whereas in a 9000-curie unit, 100 cm. SSD may be used quite comfortably because of the higher output.

Area or size of field of irradiation

The dose in a small field is attributable almost entirely to the *primary beam* (see glossary), but as the area of the field is increased, *backscatter* (see glossary) radiation is added to the primary beam, leading to increased dose. Thus, percentage depth doses increase with the area up to about 200 cm.², after which the depth dose increases much slower. The quality of the beam plays a role here also. In a 22 Mev. beam radiation scatter is negligible and so there is no difference between the depth doses of any field size.

Filter

We have discussed earlier how the addition of a filter would change the quality of the beam by removing the softer rays and letting through those of higher penetration

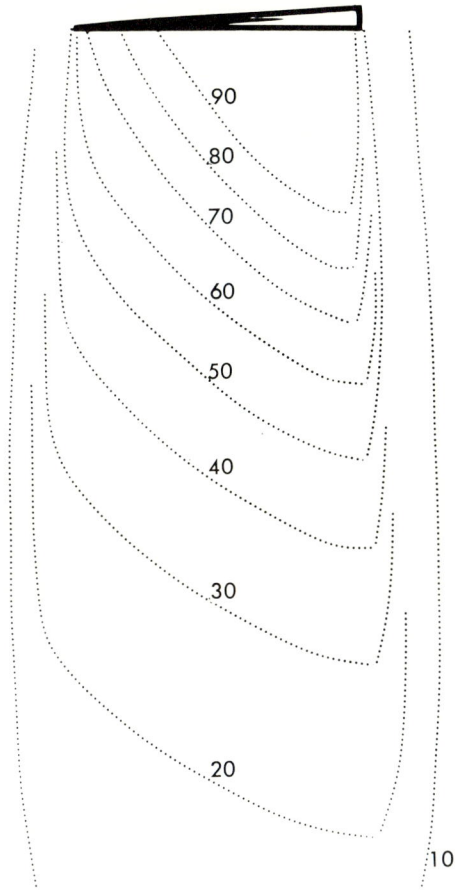

FIG. 3-9. Isodose curves of a wedge.

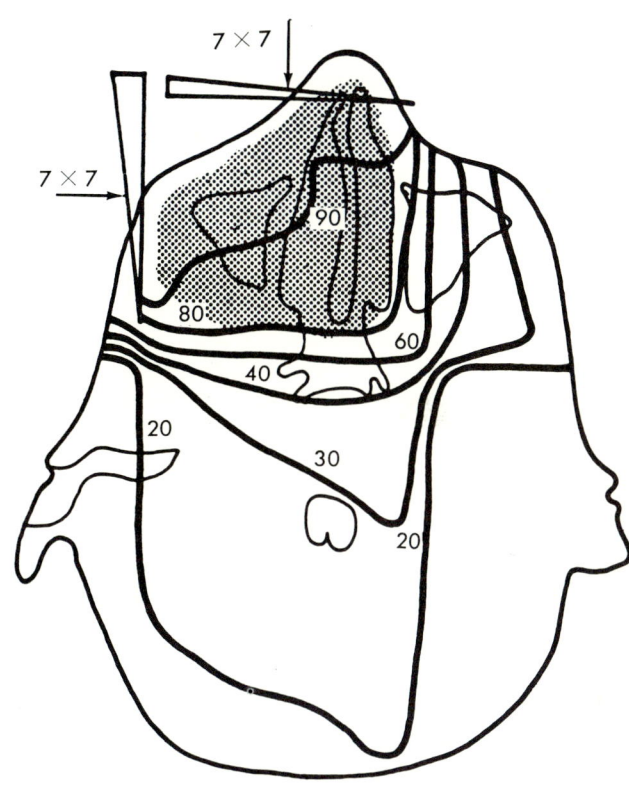

FIG. 3-10. Plan to treat an antral lesion using two wedges.

only. A special wedge lead filter has been designed for use particularly in high-voltage beams. These wedges vary in angle from 15 to 60 degrees, producing isodose curves of variable shapes, but all have the general appearance shown in Fig. 3-9. When this type of field is combined with an identical one at right angles, a region of homogeneous irradiation is produced (Fig. 3-10). Such an arrangement is ideal for the treatment of some lesions, such as laryngeal or antral carcinomas.

STEPS OF PLANNING A RADIATION THERAPY COURSE
Localizing the treatment volume

Localization films are taken while the patient is in the position of treatment, whether lying supine or prone or sitting up. This is especially important when the tumor affects a relatively mobile organ, such as a bladder. Sometimes a radiopaque material is introduced to help localization. This method is followed in a localizing cystogram in the case of a bladder carcinoma. A suitable measure is used to determine the magnification factor. X-ray films are taken in several views, with anteroposterior and lateral views being the most common.

Armed with the knowledge gained from various investigations and localization films, one may define the volume for treatment and locate it on the outline of the part to be treated taken by the aid of a pantograph. Landmarks on the outline are indicated to correspond with ones on the skin to facilitate accurate localization.

Choice of beams, fields, and doses

The first decision to be made is the choice of the *beam* to be deployed for treatment. This usually depends on the following factors:

1. *Depth of lesion.* A skin lesion may be treated successfully with a 100 to 250 kv. beam, whereas a deep lesion (such as a bronchial carcinoma) needs either a ^{60}Co unit with an 80 cm. SSD or a supervoltage x-ray beam (4 to 35 Mev.).
2. *Site of lesion.* The tumor bed, such as a lesion fixed to the bone or involving it, should be treated by either a gamma beam or a supervoltage x-ray beam to avoid excessive absorption of radiation by bone and possible complications. The same applies to a lesion involving cartilage. On the other hand, a highly penetrating beam may be harmful in the case of lesions of upper air and food passages because of the resultant high exit dose. Exit dose is the dose at the point where the axis of the beam emerges from the patient. The exit dose of a 6 Mev. beam applied laterally to the neck of an adult can reach as high as 60% depending on the thickness of the neck. Consequently, neighboring vital structures, such as larynx and spinal cord, may receive an unnecessarily high dose.
3. *Aim of treatment.* The aim of treatment, whether curative or palliative, plays a role in the choice of the equipment. For example, a palliative course aimed at treating a metastatic lesion in a femur may be carried out adequately by a 250 kv. beam, whereas a curative radical course of treatment to a reticulum cell sarcoma in the same site necessitates a supervoltage or a gamma beam (with 80 cm. SSD). Generally, when a higher dose is desired, a more penetrating beam and sophisticated plan is required.
4. *Histological diagnosis.* The histological diagnosis of the lesion plays a role in the choice of the treatment dose as well as the volume to be treated. This is discussed in greater detail in Section Three.

The next step to be decided upon is the choice of *fields or formulation of the plan of treatment.* This usually depends on the following factors:

1. *Machine chosen for treatment.*
2. *Volume to be treated.* A large volume will necessitate a different plan (Fig. 3-12) compared to a smaller volume (Fig. 3-10).
3. *Dose required.* A high dose usually necessitates a more sophisticated plan.

The final step is the *selection of the dose/time* to be used. The dose in radiotherapy must always be related to the total number of days through which it was delivered as well as the number of fractions; for example, if 6000 rads were given in 30 treatment fractions over a period of 42 days or 6 weeks, then the dose/time is expressed as 6000 rads in 42 days in 30 fractions. These three factors (total dose, number of fractions, and length of period in days) largely determine the reaction of tissues to radiation.

The dose/time delivered is largely dependent on the histological type of tumor (carcinoma versus lymphoma), the volume to be irradiated, and the objective of the treatment (radical versus palliative). These factors are discussed in more detail in Section Three.

A discussion of the various *dose definitions* used in radiation therapy is necessary: A *tumor dose* is a vague term and has no well-defined parameters. Generally, it means the dose delivered to the greater part of the treatment volume. This definition applies also to the *modal dose,* a term that is preferred by some radiotherapists. A given dose is a term usually used with single-field irradiation and is considered to be synonymous with dose maximum. For example, with radiation energy less than 300 kv., the given dose would be equal to the *skin dose* (the dose at the skin surface). For ^{60}Co irradiation the given dose would be at 5 mm. below the skin. The given dose always includes backscatter (see glossary). A *skin dose* may be useful in certain cases, such as in the case of a skin lesion treated by a 200 kv. beam or less. *Maximum tumor dose* is used to describe the maximum dose delivered to any point of significance in the tumor volume. *Minimum tumor dose* conversely means the minimum dose delivered to any point of significance. As the aim of every radiotherapist is to deliver homogeneous dose to the volume treated, the difference between the maximum and minimum dose must be kept to a minimum. A *homogeneous dose* within the treated volume ensures two very important points—first, that all the tumor receives the dose aimed at to accomplish the objectives of the treatment and, second, to avoid overirradiation and damage to surrounding normal tissues. A *midpoint dose* is the term usually used when two opposing fields are employed to indicate the dose at a midway plane. The *integral dose* is used to describe the total energy absorbed by the patient from the beam used in treatment. It does not necessarily reflect the dose given to the tumor. It depends on various factors: (1) Type of beam. Generally the more penetrating the beam, the higher the integral dose. However, there are few exceptions to this general law. (2) Size of the fields applied. The larger the fields applied, the higher the integral dose. (3) The number of the fields applied. The more numerous the fields, the higher the integral dose. However, if some of the fields are filtered by a wedge or if parts of the fields are shielded, then the integral dose is reduced. It is highly desirable to keep the integral dose as low as possible to diminish the general effect of radiation.

It would be appropriate here to define the *units of radiation* which are used—the roentgen, the rad, and the ret.

The *roentgen* is defined as an exposure dose of x or gamma radiation such that the associated corpuscular emission (ions of either charge) per 0.001293 gram of air produces, in air, ions carrying one electrostatic unit of quantity of electricity of either sign. The quantity of 0.001293 gram of air is the mass of 1 cm.^{3} of dry air at normal temperature and pressure (760 mm. of mercury pressure at 0° C.). To measure a dose in roentgens, one must segregate (in a chamber) a known mass of air and measure the ionization in this air. Such a device is called an *ionization chamber*. The roentgen (*R*, not *r*) is essentially a unit of exposure dose. It was first adopted by the International Congress of Radiology held in Stockholm in 1928. It is more important to the radiotherapist to know the dose absorbed by the patient rather than the dose of radiation that emerges from a machine. Generally for x-ray or gamma beams of less than 3 Mev. energy, the roentgen may be used to measure the absorbed dose, but it is impossible to use it for x-ray beams of energy higher than 3 Mev. or for particle beams (electrons, deuterons). That is why another unit was adopted as a unit of absorbed radiation and was called the rad.

The rad corresponds to an energy absorption of 100 ergs per gram (see glossary). The erg is a unit of energy. The rad is defined in terms of energy, since the radiotherapist is interested in the amount of energy absorbed by tissues because this will be reflected in the biological effects of radiation.

To convert roentgens into rads, one uses a conversion factor *(f)*. This factor *f* has been calculated for different energies and different tissues as shown below:

Energy (Mev.)	*f*	
	Muscle	Bone
0.01	0.933	3.58
0.1	0.957	1.47
1	0.974	0.965

Since most radiation beams contain a spectrum of photon energies, the values of

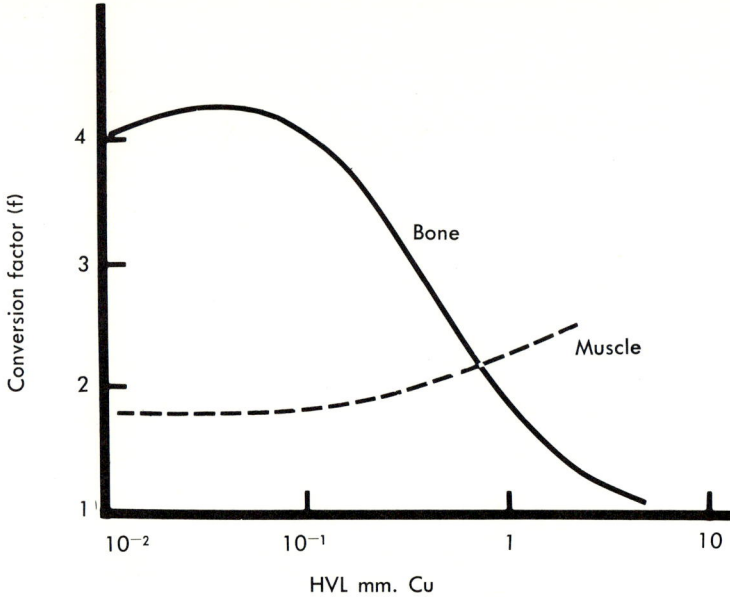

Fig. 3-11. Conversion factors of muscle and bone.

f must be averaged over the spectrum. This has been done, and the results are shown in Fig. 3-11 where the conversion factors are plotted against the half-value layer (which expresses the quality of the beam) for muscle and bone. The factor for bone falls from over 4.3 to 1.1 as the half-value layer is increased from 0.01 to 4 mm. of copper. Over the same range, the value for muscle increases from 0.93 to 0.97. This confirms, in a mathematical fashion, what was discussed earlier: the higher the energy of the beam, the more homogeneous is the absorption in bone and muscle.

Field arrangements

The plans formulated to treat any lesion are unique to this lesion in its circumstances; that is why discussion of all details here is impossible. However, after the following outline it would be appropriate to discuss a few representative arrangements:

1. *Fixed-field techniques*
   a. Two opposing fields (Fig. 3-12)
   b. Three open fields (Fig. 3-13)
   c. Two wedge fields (Fig. 3-10)
   d. Three fields (one open and two wedges) (Fig. 3-14)
   e. Four fields (4 wedges) (Fig. 3-15)
2. *Rotation therapy*

Fixed-field techniques

Two opposing fields (Fig. 3-12). This is the most commonly used combination of fields, which may be either anterior and posterior or alternatively right and left lateral. The setting of the patient is very simple, especially in the presence of an accurate back pointer (see p. 46). The resultant radiation affects the section of the body under treatment homogeneously within a certain volume. However, there may be two areas of relatively increased intensity corresponding to the fields of entry, especially if the separation between the two opposing fields is relatively large. With such large separation there is also a falloff at the edge of the beam in the middle of the treatment volume (a so-called waist). The two main disadvantages of using two opposing fields are (1) that there is a relatively high skin dose (en-

Planning of radiotherapy treatment 41

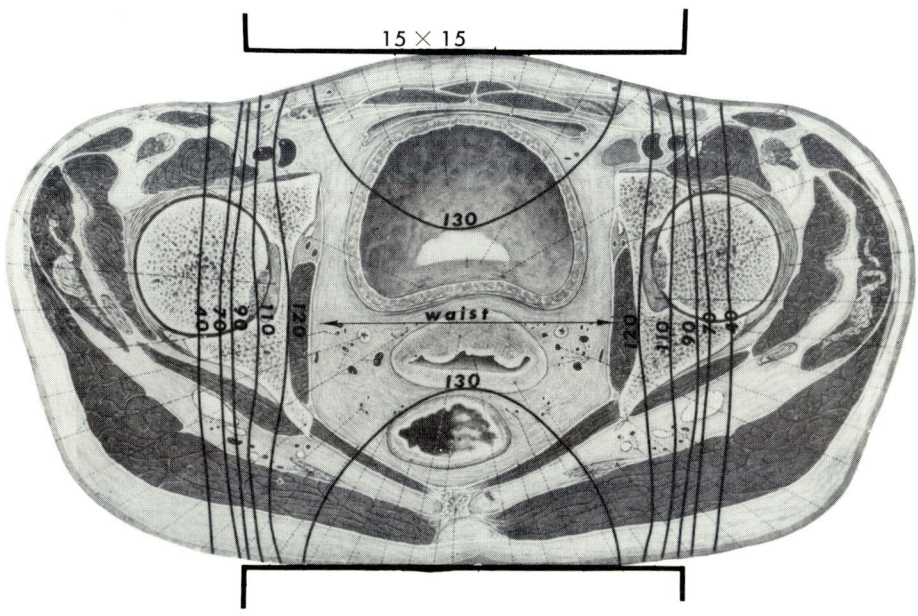

FIG. 3-12. Plan of treatment of whole pelvis using two opposed fields.

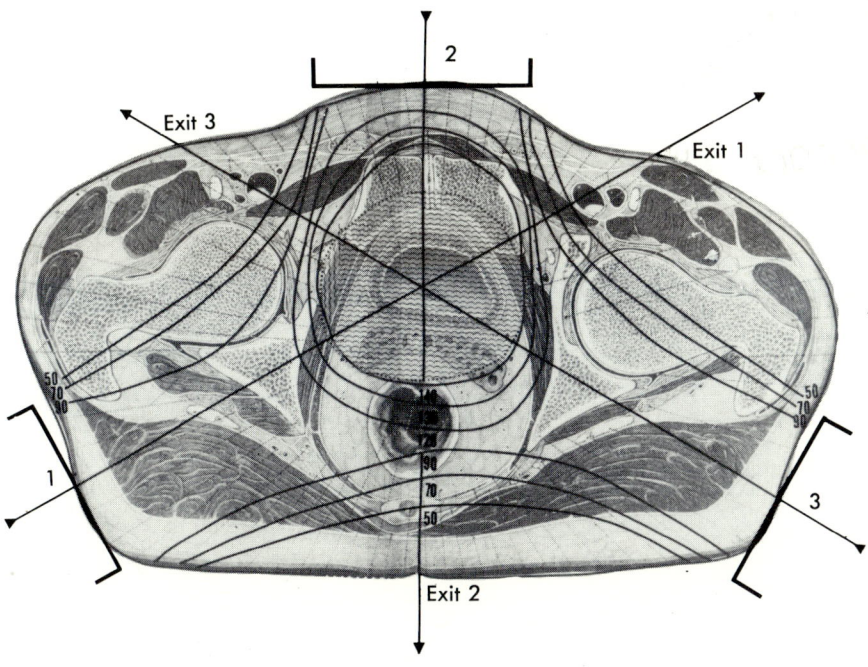

FIG. 3-13. Plan of treatment of a bladder lesion using three open fields.

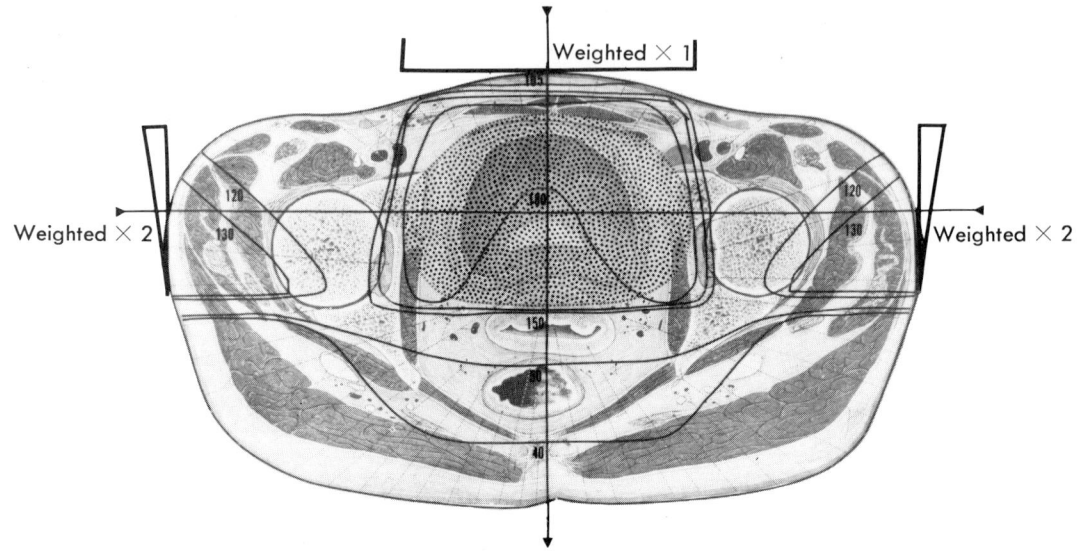
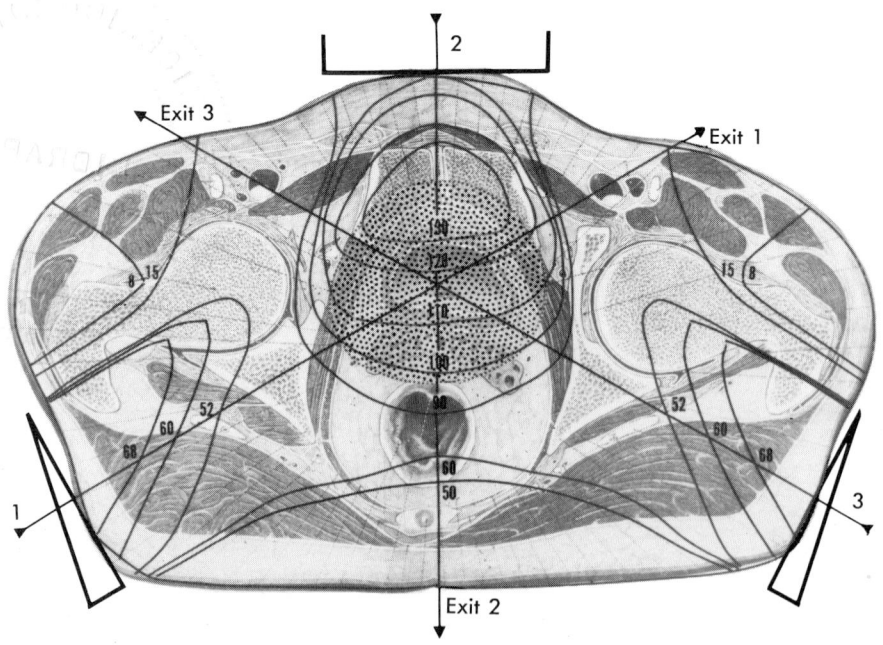

Fig. 3-14. Plan to treat bladder and perivesical tissues using one open field (anterior) and two lateral wedges.

trance and exit dose), especially when the separation between the two fields is rather small and (2) that the whole treated section of the body receives the full dose without discrimination or protection to important normal structures (such as the spinal cord). This plan is suited to treat large volumes to moderate doses (malignant lymphomas) or a large volume without the need of protection to any surrounding structure (a sarcomatous lesion in a limb).

Three and four open fields plan. The term "open fields" means 'unwedged.' Combinations of three or four open fields are used to treat various shaped volumes. The two main factors that dictate the number of fields are the depth of the tumor (generally the deeper the tumor, the more fields needed) and the quality of the beam (the less penetrating the beam is, the more fields needed).

Two-wedge plan. If two 45-degree wedges are positioned perpendicularly to each other, the resultant isodose curves form a regular diamond (Fig. 3-10) because of the particular shape of the isodose curves of the wedge field (Fig. 3-9). However, if the angle of the wedge changes or both wedges are not placed perpendicularly to each other, the resultant diamond will have a different shape. By changing these two factors, one can treat variable shaped volumes and protect any vital struture.

Combinations of wedge and open fields. Combinations of wedge and open fields increase the versatility of the planning, and it is possible to treat almost any volume to a high dose with a very high degree of protection to wherever it is needed. Fig. 13-1 (two wedge fields and one open field) exemplifies this fact, whereby it is possible to treat a kidney (or a kidney bed) and the neighboring para-aortic lymph nodes with enough protection to the spinal cord (to keep its dose within tolerance) and almost complete protection to the other kidney nearby.

Some general snags in the planning of

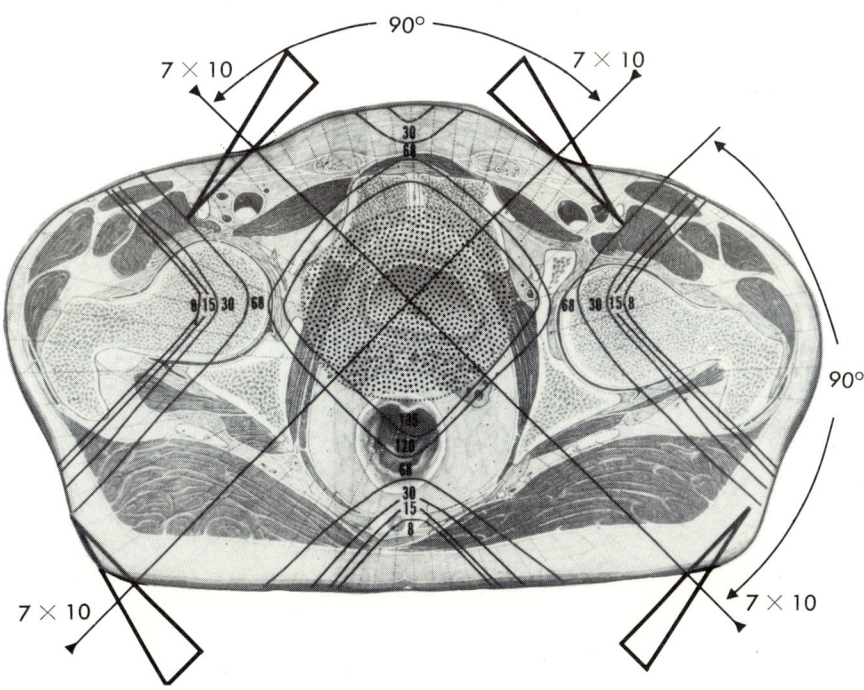

Fig. 3-15. Plan to treat bladder using four wedge fields.

composite fields are discussed in the following paragraphs.

BODY INHOMOGENEITY. As mentioned earlier, the isodose curves used in planning have generally been plotted in a water medium, but the body is not all that homogeneous, since it is formed of layers of soft tissue (muscles, fasciae, fat), bone, with its special absorption faculties, and cavities, such as lungs and paranasal sinuses. When high-energy beams are generally used for planning, bone does not present particular problems, but air cavities do, especially if they are traversed to a substantial length, such as in treating some cases of the middle third of esophageal carcinoma. If no corrections are made, the tumor dose may be undercalculated by about 20%. In such cases, necessary corrections should be carried out to avoid overdosage. This will depend mainly on the thickness of tissues traversed and the particular energy used.

CURVATURE OF THE BODY SURFACE. When the isodose curves were plotted, all the treatment rays hit the surface at equal points (because the surface of the water phantom is flat). Because most of the body surfaces are curves, this situation is bound to affect the dose distribution in the body. Should the curves be of such dimensions that the changes are of significance (such as those of the breast), then this curvature should be either corrected (by using a bolus) or taken into consideration in the calculation (to achieve a correct dose). Bolus is a packed material that is built up on a curved body surface to produce a flat surface instead of the curve. The result will be more homogeneous dose absorption. Bolus is made of any material whose absorption characteristics are similar to tissue. Wax and special rice bags are the material most commonly used. However, bolus is not without disadvantages. The main one is the loss of the skin-sparing effect of the high-energy beam. The bolus being placed against the skin pulls the maximum buildup of the dose to the surface of the skin instead of below the skin.

Rotation therapy. In all the previous field arrangements both the patient and the machine are fixed during treatment (fixed-field techniques). In rotation therapy, however, either the patient or the machine are in movement during treatment. The advantages of such a technique are mainly simplicity in setting up where the machine is set to one point (point of entry of the beam along the central axis of rotation) at a fixed distance, which is the source-to-tumor distance, D. However, since a deep tumor is not visible, the distance between the skin and the center of the tumor, F (or treated volume), and the source-to-skin distance, S, which is used to set the patient, is calculated as follows:

$$S = D - F$$

Another advantage of this technique is the ability to deliver a high tumor dose to the tumor with a much smaller amount of radiation to the surrounding tissues (Fig. 3-16). Rotation may be either *complete*, for a full 360 degrees, or only *partial*, for a fraction of the 360-degree circumference. Another form of rotation is *arc therapy*, whereby the machine moves in a manner akin to a clock pendulum.

The main parameter used to assess the dose to tumor or tissue in rotation is the tumor-air ratio, R (or tissue-air ratio), which represents the ratio between the dose at the depth of the tumor, D_t, as related to the dose at the same depth had there been no intervening tissue, D_{ta}, with a simple equation:

$$R = \frac{D_t}{D_{ta}}$$

This ratio behaves in a manner similar to the depth dose previously discussed; that is, both are dependent on the depth of the tumor (Fig. 3-7), the area of the field, and the quality of the beam. An example of the resultant isodose curves in rotational therapy is shown in Fig. 3-16. Another factor that may affect these curves is the beam

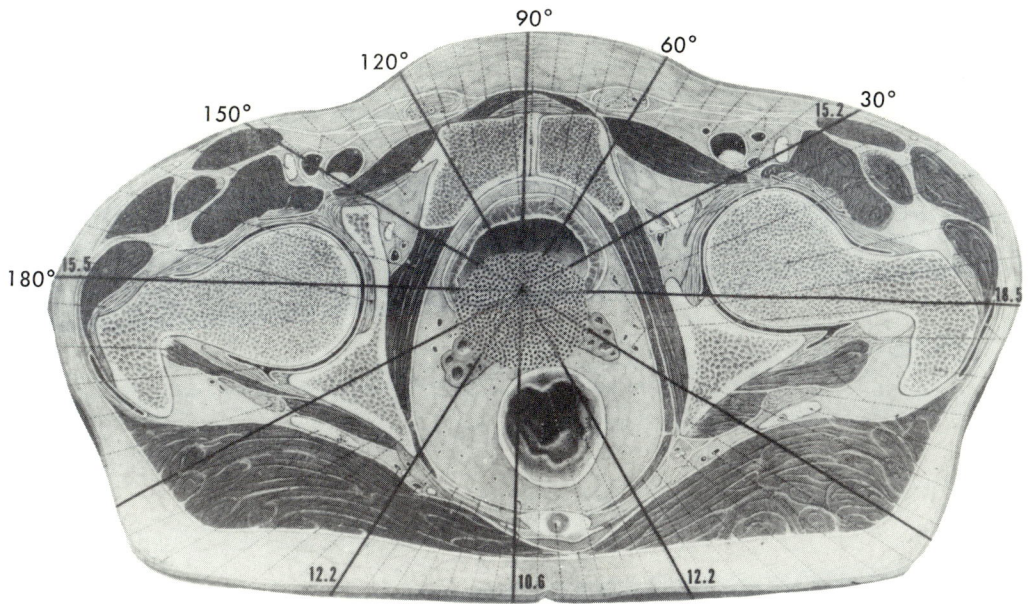

Fig. 3-16. Plan for treatment of a prostatic lesion with rotation. The following table shows the calculation of a tumor dose in rotation (d, thickness of tissues; $T.M.R$, ratio between dose at center and maximum dose):

ANGLE	DISTANCE = d	TISSUE MAXIMUM RATIOS
0°	18.5	0.490
30°	15.2	0.577
60°	11	0.705
90°	10	0.732
120°	10.5	0.722
150°	12.5	0.657
180°	15.5	0.569
210°	17.5	0.516
240°	12.2	0.667
270°	10.6	0.721
300°	12.2	0.667
330°	21.5	0.424

Tumor dose calculated 62%

penumbra, because the smaller the penumbra, the better the distribution.

The ideal distribution of these curves is where they form circles with maximum intensity around the volume to be treated, with a rapid falloff in the surrounding normal tissues. Unfortunately this is not always possible and very often surrounding tissues receive a relatively high dose, such as in the lungs in case of the treatment of esophageal carcinoma. This is the main limiting factor in rotation therapy.

Checking the treatment plan

Checking, as the last step, is very important before the plan is put in action. It is aimed at (1) ensuring the fact that the treatment volume is in fact the tumor-bearing volume and (2) ensuring the applicability of the plan (as drawn on paper) to the treatment volume. Since shielding is often employed to protect normal body structures, it is important to check on this aspect also. With the high-energy beams, which are commonly in use nowadays, mar-

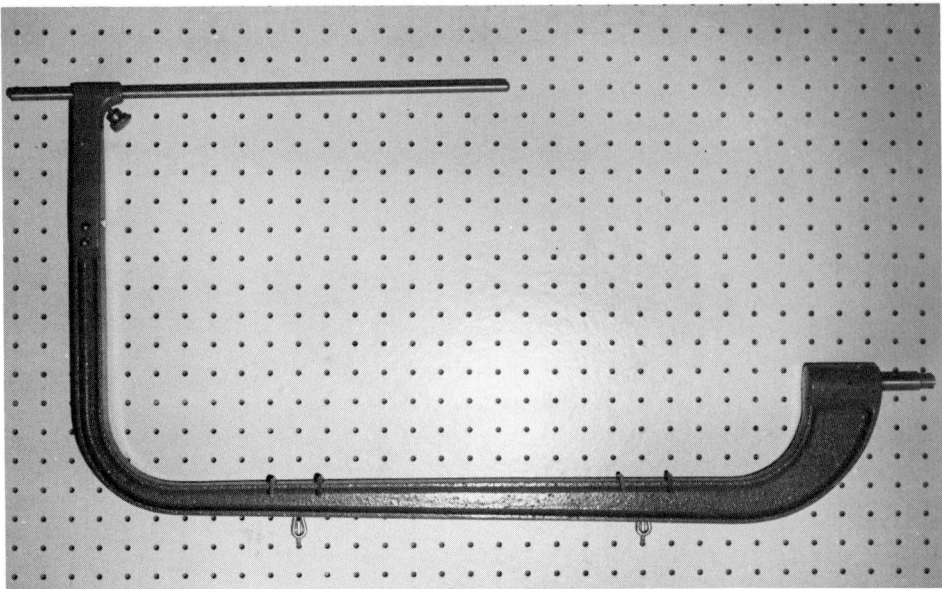

Fig. 3-17. Mechanical back pointer.

ginal errors may be very harmful. The various methods used to achieve these objectives are by back pointers, use of check films, direct measurements, and reproducing plans on phantoms, discussed as follows.

Back pointers. These are either mechanical devices (Fig. 3-17) or a light beam arrangement. When a patient is located in front of the treatment beam, the back point represents the exit point of the beam. Thus, when these two points are accurately marked, the device using it ensures that the tumor is always located in the treatment volume.

Use of check films. These films should be obtained on the simulator while the patient is set in exactly the same treatment position (with the same Perspex cast when used). The diagnostic beam is set at exactly the same source-to-skin distance used in treatment with the same angles. Landmarks and some opaque material (such as cystogram or opaque material in the balloon of a Foley catheter) may be used to help identify the treatment volume. Check films may also be obtained on the treatment unit itself (by use of the treatment beam). The disadvantage of such a film is its poor diagnostic quality. Under a high-energy beam, bones are not easily distinguishable from soft tissues (because of similar absorption characteristics); usual opaque materials, such as barium sulfate in the esophagus or diatrizoate sodium (Hypaque Sodium) in the bladder, are similarly unidentifiable, but air cavities stand out in good contrast (that is, in a ^{60}Co beam). Other radiopaque materials may be used to overcome this problem, such as mercury, which is injected into the balloon of a Foley catheter (Fig. 3-18).

Direct measurements. This is one of the best methods to check any treatment plan. It consists of introducing special dosimeters, such as ionization chambers or thermoluminescent dosimeters, into the volume to be treated and getting a direct measurement of the actual dose delivered during treatment. Unfortunately, this method is only applicable in certain sites, such as in esophageal carcinoma by introduction of

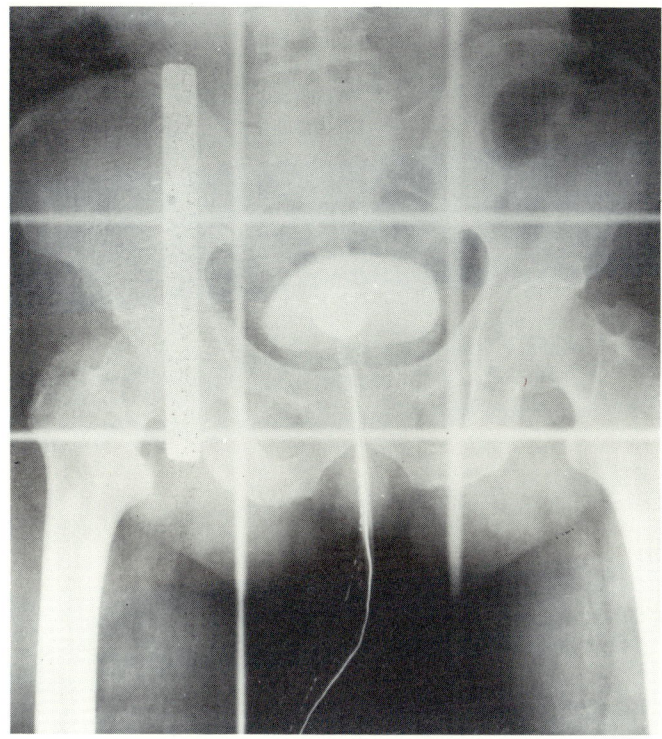

Fig. 3-18. Check film of treatment of prostate with mercury injected into a balloon of a Foley catheter and dye in bladder.

the dosimeter into the esophagus; vaginal lesions; rectal carcinoma; and lesions of the oral cavity or nose. Sometimes it is possible to measure the dose to a neighboring vital structure, such as the eye in the case of treatment of a paranasal lesion.

Reproducing a plan of treatment on a phantom. This method is rather complicated and used only in case of organs deeply situated in the body. Moreover, it is possible only to check a general plan to treat a certain site (and not a specific case). A representative body phantom is used, such as the Rando phantom (Fig. 3-4) whereby the relevant section of the body is identified and an ideal plan of treatment has evolved. The following three methods are available to check on such a plan and get direct measurements.

1. In the *film method*, a film is placed between the layers of the phantom during treatment. This exposed film is then scanned in a densitometer so that the different densities on the film (which represents different levels of dose) can be measured and recorded.

2. *Special ionization chambers* are inserted into predrilled holes in each section of the phantom, and the absorbed dose is measured after exposure to the therapy beam. The obvious disadvantage of this system is that doses are measured in a phantom and not directly in a patient.

3. The *thermoluminescent dosimeter* (TLD) is usually made up of crystals of either magnesium fluoride or lithium fluoride, which responds when irradiated in an unusual manner; they appear unaffected although they store energy. When heated, the irradiated crystals release the stored energy as light. The total amount of light measured by a photomultiplier instrument

is roughly proportional to the dosage to which the crystals were exposed. The crystals come in the form of disks (1 cm. in diameter), rods (1 mm. in diameter), and powder. These forms make them usable in almost any kind of body cavity.

SECTION TWO

BIOLOGICAL EFFECTS OF RADIATION

The following chapter summarizes the biological effects of radiation on the human organism, as pertaining to cell, tissue (a complex cellular structure), organ (a complex tissue structure), and the total organism (a complex of organs). A word of warning—the concepts and measurements of radiation effects are sometimes vague because of the body's complex structure, the interdependence of various organ systems, and the body's homeostatic mechanism. For example, the dysfunction caused by damage of a certain tissue would depend, among other factors, on the type of tissue and how vital it is to the organism (contrast nervous tissue versus connective tissue), the extent of the damage, the ability of the tissue to restore itself, and the existence of a compensatory mechanism. An attempt at relating cellular damage to subsequent organ function has been carried out; similarly organ and total body changes have been related. However, as vagueness may mark such a trial, you may come to appreciate the complexity of the problem.

CHAPTER 4

EFFECTS OF RADIATION ON CELLS

INTERFERENCE WITH MITOSIS

Fig. 4-1 shows the basic structure of the cell. The experience with radiation over the last 50 years has shown that the dramatic changes produced by radiation in tissues are related to interference with mitosis. Fig. 4-2 shows the various stages of cellular division or mitosis—prophase, metaphase, anaphase, and telophase. During the *prophase* dense filaments appear in the nucleus. The newly recognized filaments gradually become shorter and form spiral structures. They are composed of two threads known as the chromatids. During the *metaphase* the nuclear membrane disappears, and a protein fibrous structure called the *spindle* appears in the cytoplasm. The spindle extends to the opposite poles of the cell. The polypeptide chains run parallel to the axis of the spindle and perpendicular to the equatorial plate in the center of the cell where the chromosomes assemble. Each chromosome attaches itself to a fiber of the spindle at a single point, the centromere, where the chromosomes are usually bent.

During the *anaphase,* the chromosomes divide and the chromatids separate in the region of the centromeres to form daughter chromosomes. These move toward the opposite poles of the cell along the spindle and result in an equal number of chromosomes at each end.

During the *telophase* the chromosomes fuse back to a fine network of chromatin, which eventually becomes invisible while a nuclear membrane reforms around it. The cellular cytoplasm is divided into two approximately equal parts by a new cellular membrane, which completes the formation of two daughter cells, which are assumed to contain the same cytoplasmic structures of the original cell, that is, the mitochondria.

All cells except the gametes or reproductive cells (sperm and ovum) multiply ultimately by mitosis to form tissues. The sperm and the ovum are formed by meiosis, which differs in some respects from mitosis. Meiosis consists of two successive cellular divisions in which the chromosome complement is only duplicated once, such that each gamete carries only half the usual number of chromosomes. The original num-

52 *Biological effects of radiation*

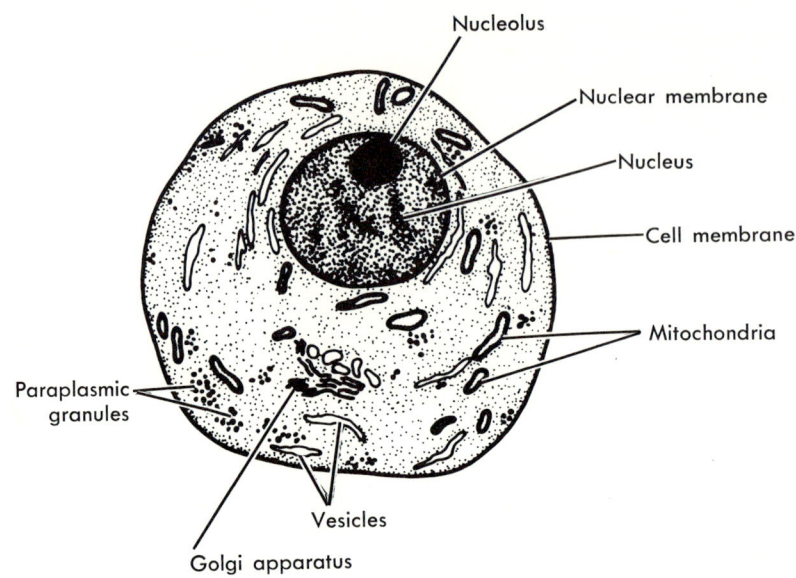

FIG. 4-1. Diagram of main cellular structures.

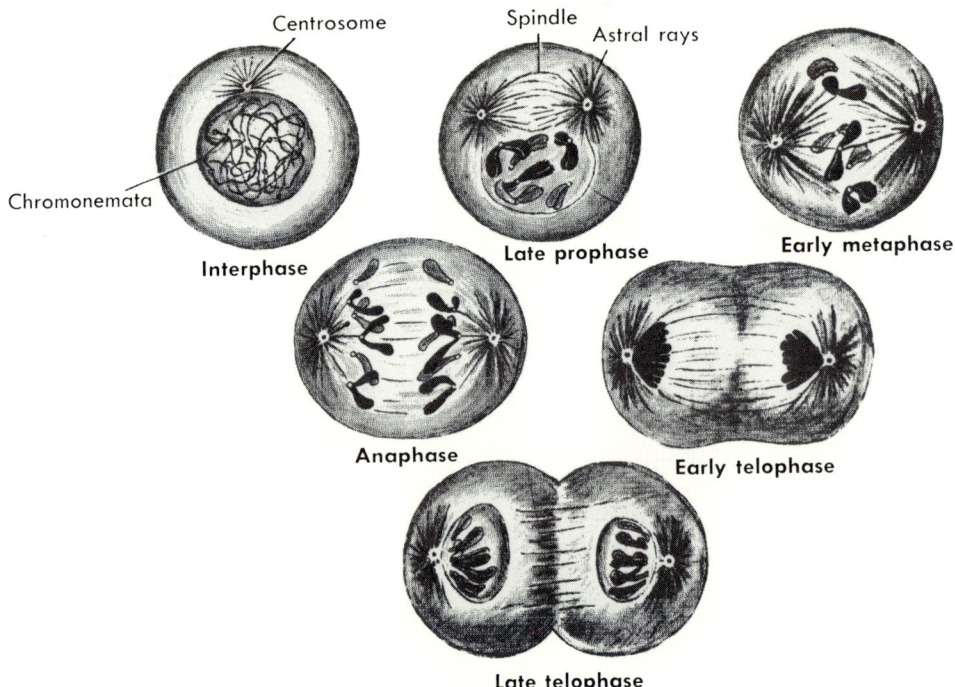

FIG. 4-2. Changes that occur in the process of mitotic division.

ber is reestablished by fusion of the gametes. Not all cells divide at a regular pace. In a mammal like man cells of certain tissues never divide, such as the neurons (of the central nervous system), some divide rarely, such as the liver, whereas others are continuously dividing, such as the deep layer of epidermis, bone marrow, or crypts of intestinal epithelia.

The study of the effects of radiation on mitosis has led early radiologists (Bergonié and Tribondeau) to formulate their famous law "the sensitivity of cells to irradiation is in direct proportion to their reproductive activity and inversely proportional to their degree of differentiation." Although this law correctly predicts the effect of radiation on mitosis as studied in tissue cultures, clinical facts in radiation therapy do not always support it; for example, highly undifferentiated carcinomas are not necessarily radiosensitive and rapidly growing embryonal sarcomas are known to be relatively radioresistant.

Taking these limitations into consideration the changes in mitosis caused by radiation are classified into the following two stages.

Delay in the onset of mitosis followed by a normal mitosis. Such an incident indicates that there was a certain degree of cell damage that was restored completely. This usually happens when a small dose is given before the prophase (before the start of the mitosis). The mechanism of such a delay may be a result of damage to some mechanism that controls the onset of mitosis (or the maintenance of growth). However, certain authors claim that such an incident is linked with inhibition of DNA synthesis.

Complete inhibition of mitosis where the cell continues to live and function or metabolizes but is completely unable to divide. Such sterile cells may represent the so-called sterile residual malignant disease that may be seen after radiotherapy. Examination of such residual disease under the microscope would reveal viable cells, but such cells would be incapable of local growth or metastatic deposits. Unfortunately there is no way to differentiate microscopically between sterile cells and cells capable of dividing.

CELL DEATH

There are three types of the degree of injury called cell death—mitotic or genetic death, interphase death, and instant death.

Cell death after one or more divisions have occurred is called *mitotic or genetic death*. It occurs in general with doses smaller than are needed to produce interphase death (see below) in cells that no longer divide or that divide only very slowly. The cells may either degenerate after one or two (or a few) divisions or form a giant cell in tissue cultures. The giant cell does not divide but continues to synthesize nucleic acids (DNA and RNA) and to grow to huge sizes (hence the name giant) though eventually it degenerates.

In both cases the cells are unable to form macroscopic colonies in tissue culture. Such effects are found by Puck to occur after an exposure dose of as little as 75 R. At higher doses even single cell division is precluded, but a large proportion of these cells give rise to giants. It appears that giant cell formation is the most common result of cellular damage in this phase.

Other authors claim different quantitative dose effects. Kohn and Fogh believed that a dose of 600 R. merely delays division and only with doses of 1000 R. did cells start to degenerate. One must remember that these results were found in tissue culture, where the cells are more or less isolated. In the human body different cells lie in a state of adherence to surrounding cellular structures, which exercise a definite modifying effect. Thus there is a large difference that exists, on occasions, between in vivo (in human beings) and in vitro (in laboratory test tube or tissue culture plate) studies.

Cell death occurring many hours after irradiation, but without there being any intervening division, is called *interphase death*. It occurs when irradiation dose is sufficiently high to cause depolymerization of DNA, resulting in progressive destruction of the nucleus. Concomitantly, the morphology of the nucleoli may also be altered as evidenced by fragmentation and vacuolation. The doses required to produce these changes vary greatly from cell to cell, with the sensitive ones (lymphocytes, spermatogonia) killed by a few hundred rads whereas less sensitive ones (cells in bones) may require several thousand rads. It is for this type of cell death that the law of Bergonié and Tribondeau has the widest validity.

Instant death usually occurs after very high doses of the order of 100,000 rads, which would coagulate many cellular proteins. In practical radiotherapy, death of the cells from radiation damage inflicted during mitosis plays a minor role in the treatment of malignant tumors. This is so because malignant tumor cells have a much longer life-span than do normal cells. That is why radiotherapy exercises its successful effect mostly either by an interphase death or by sterilizing the cell.

BREAKAGE OF CHROMOSOMES

Cells are most sensitive to chromosome breakage when irradiated during interphase. The damage is only seen at metaphase or anaphase. Cells irradiated during mitosis show permanent chromosome abnormalities in subsequent mitotic cycles but not in the same mitosis. Two changes are assumed to occur—the severing of the chromosome by direct effect of radiation and then the rejoining of the fragments, producing new configurations, provided that no excessive time lag interval exists (only a few minutes). These changes are highly dose-rate dependent. Some chemotherapeutic drugs also may lead to the same effect (called mutation). Moreover these mutations are qualitatively the same as those that occur naturally.

Some of the changes produced in chromosomes can be reproduced in their following divisions and thus become perpetuated. Since chromosomes carry genes, permanent structural changes may result in *genetic changes*. Genes determine heritable characters and are formed of deoxyribonucleic acid (DNA) in association with proteins. They are located at specific points within the chromosomes.

Since mutations may occur naturally, it is important to compare the rate of a given mutation in any organism after irradiation, to the naturally occurring rate. A term used for this is the "doubling dose." The doubling dose is the dose of ionizing radiation that when given in a single exposure doubles the natural rate of a given mutation. It is almost impossible to determine accurately the doubling dose in human beings, since, obviously, no such human experimentation is possible. However, there are a few accepted assumptions regarding the mutagenic effects of radiation on human beings: the effect of the dose given is cumulative and it takes a long time, sometimes generations, for detection of such an effect. Mutations are not restricted to germ cells (genetic effect) but also occur in somatic cells (somatic mutations). This is not unexpected, since DNA-containing nucleoproteins exist in all cells and are identical in quality in both germ and somatic cells. Leukemia and cancer induced after irradiation exposure are considered to be the result of such somatic mutations.

IMPAIRMENT OF FUNCTION WITHOUT CELL DEATH

This is especially manifest in differentiated and specialized cells when the dose of irradiation is sublethal (see glossary). The resultant damage depends on the particular cell. For example, leukocytes lose their phagocytic activity, respiratory epithelial cells lose their ciliary motion, and secretory cells like those of salivary gland or gastric mucosa suffer from impaired activity.

The effect of such cellular damage on the whole tissue or indeed on the whole organism is also damaging and can be profound especially in the case of highly specialized secretory cells like those of the thyroid or the pituitary gland. Hypothyroidism and diabetes insipidus are examples of such damage. Details of these damages are discussed at length in the following paragraphs under the appropriate tissue headings.

CHAPTER 5

EFFECT OF RADIATION ON TISSUES

In the preceding chapter we discussed the effect of radiation at the cellular level. The findings depended largely on radiological experiments with tissue culture or experimental animals. The findings that are described in the following paragraphs are largely dependent on clinical and histological observation in humans and, as such, are much more relevant to practical radiotherapy.

Although the effects of radiation on various tissues are basically similar, tissue sensitivity and function vary so much that it is advantageous to discuss each tissue separately. However, three salient facts apply to the radiation damage of all tissues:

1. It depends on the dose-time factor, that is, the dose given as related to the total time interval during which this dose was applied (measured in total number of rads in total number of days).
2. The larger the volume irradiated, the more pronounced is the damage. The term "volume" is used deliberately instead of "portal of entry," since the volume depends on such important factors as the quality of the beam, and the number and arragement of the fields (or portals of entry) employed.
3. Dose rate, that is, the number of rads delivered in a unit of time (minute or second), may play a role in determining tissue sensitivity.

SKIN

Skin is the tissue most commonly affected by radiation whether treatment is specifically directed to it (such as in a skin lesion) or directed to an internal lesion (such as a bladder carcinoma). In the early days of radiotherapy when beams used for external radiotherapy were limited to energies below 250 kv., skin changes were so consistent that they were used for measuring the dose of radiation given (for erythema dose, see glossary). With the advent of supervoltage beams and cobalt beams where the buildup of the maximum dose is deep to the skin, such changes lost their significance and importance. In addition to the factors that affect radiation damage mentioned earlier (beam quality, dose-time applied, and volume irradiated) the particular site of the skin irradiated is of some importance: for example, the skin areas of the perineum, buttock, and retromammary sulcus are known for their relatively poor radiation tolerance. This poor tolerance is attributable more to the presence of excessive moisture and warmth in these regions rather than to the tissue per se. Gross radiation damage to the skin is summarized as follows: patchy erythematous reaction where the skin becomes red and florid followed by a confluent erythema. The time factor varies (according to the above discussion) up to 48 hours for the early reaction and up to about 14 days for the late ones.

Should the radiation insult continue, edema and moist desquamation occur, leaving a raw surface akin to a second-degree burn. A further stage of damage would involve destruction of both dermis and epidermis (similar to a third-degree burn): such damage should not be encountered in radiation therapy under usual circumstances. The edema that accompanies the radiation-induced skin damage may persist for weeks or months, with the excess fluid firmly bound and incorporated in swollen, degenerated collagen and elastic tissue.

The *skin appendages* are also destroyed, resulting in temporary epilation when the dose is of the order of a few hundred rads. Permanent epilation occurs with higher doses. However, it varies according to the energy used. This dose is higher in the case of supervoltage or cobalt beams than that of the 250 kv. beam, since the site of maximum buildup of the dose is deeper than that of the hair follicle. Epilation in the head and neck region occurs in areas consistent with the beam (^{60}Co or supervoltage) exit point because of a relatively high exit dose (see glossary). After temporary epilation the regenerated hair may change quality (curly versus straight) or color. Loss of function of sweat and sebaceous glands occur along the same lines.

The healing process of skin takes about 3 weeks and sometimes several weeks or months to be completed, depending on the degree of destruction. If the dose was moderate, florid erythema progresses to dusky erythema and then to dry desquamation in about 6 weeks and finally complete healing 3 to 4 weeks later. However, sometimes the area of reaction may be permanently marked with a slight tan. Although this skin is grossly and microscopically normal, its tolerance to further radiation (x rays or sun rays) is greatly reduced.

If the damage was severe, the process of healing is somewhat different. Edema is succeeded by a permanent type of hard or "woody" edema as coarse bundles of collagen are laid down. Blood vessels are permanently hyalinized and obstructed and leave either a clear scar or atrophic skin, which is tense, shiny, and dry. There may be regular areas of pigmentation or depigmentation. Spiderlike ramifications of telangiectatic vessels appear. Skin appendages (hair, sweat, and sebaceous glands) either disappear completely or persist in a rudimentary nonfunctional state. Such skin is prone to cracking or ulceration under any insult (thermal, physical). Radiation ulcers and carcinomas of the skin may sometimes occur many years after such incidents.

The principles of *treatment* of skin reaction are similar to the management of skin burns of the same severity. Erythematous skin should be kept dry and well aerated. The application of a powder (like baby powders or corn starch) may lessen the itching, which can be bothersome on occasions. For moist desquamation the application of an antibiotic ointment, in addition to an ointment containing vitamins A and D, seems to speed healing. Mild antiseptics like gentian violet or dilute solutions of hydrogen peroxide may be used if the area affected is small.

MUCOUS MEMBRANE

Mucous membranes line the gastrointestinal tract as well as the upper respiratory system including the trachea and bronchi. Although radiation changes in all sites are basically the same, the tolerance varies from one site to the other. Mucous membrane of the intestines is known for its radiosensitivity (and sensitivity to cytotoxic agents), which would explain why diarrhea and intestinal mucous-membrane ulcerations are among the early changes after whole-body or large abdominal field irradiation. Oral mucous membrane as well as that of the rectum and respiratory system has a relatively better tolerance. Even in the oral cavity itself various areas are more tolerant than are others. The dorsum of the tongue, the base of the tongue, and the cheek have a better tolerance than do the soft palate and the floor of the mouth.

The first radiation-induced change to the mucous membrane is usually functional. There is a change of taste in the case of oral epithelium or a loss of ciliary function in the case of the respiratory system. These changes occur in the first 2 weeks of a radiotherapy course. Congestion and loss of the normal glistening smoothness of the membrane represent the early anatomical changes. This is accompanied by further interference with normal function, such as hoarseness of voice. A second degree of radiation damage is mucositis, which is followed by the formation of a thin whitish film, or false membrane as it is sometimes called. Mucositis may lead to several symptoms, such as noticeable soreness if the mucous membrane treated is in sensitive areas, like the oral cavity. Motor dysfunction is another sequela, such as dysphagia or colics in the case of the motile parts of the alimentary canal (esophagus or intestines). Diarrhea is a very common symptom at this stage if large bowels or rectum are the regions affected.

These changes occur early in intestinal mucous membrane and lead to serious diarrhea and tenesmus. If the segment of intestines irradiated is unduly large or if the insult is excessive, such a reaction can be very serious and may indeed prove to be fatal. If radiation is delivered slowly over a relatively long time, the second level of reaction (mucositis and membrane formation) is rarely encountered. The mucous membrane is characterized by relatively rapid healing compared to the skin. If the radiation insult was moderate, the resultant mucous membrane after healing is of normal character, whereas the membrane is usually atrophic with areas of telangiectasia if the reaction was excessive. Atrophic mucous membrane may be tender if it is situated in sensitive areas like the oral cavity and may be a source of continuous irritation and pain. It may also lead to permanent functional derangements in certain sites, such as the vocal cords where the voice can be permanently impaired (hoarseness), or the esophagus where atrophy or stenosis may lead to continuing difficulty in swallowing. Incidents whereby patients died from inanition because of a complete inability to swallow after an esophageal cancer had been extinguished are not unknown. This is especially common if tumors occur in areas where the esophagus is anatomically narrowed.

The *appendages* of the mucous membrane—the serous glands—are very prone to radiation damage. This is usually noticed during the fourth week of irradiation, that is, after a dose of about 3000 rads. The earliest change is usually thickening of the secretions (such as the saliva, resulting in a sensation of the dryness of mouth). Higher doses will lead to a similar damage of the mucous glands, resulting in increasing dryness of the mucous membrane. These changes interfere with the function of the alimentary tract. If the damage occurs in the oral cavity, it results in a dry food bolus, which is difficult to masticate and swallow. Secondary infections, such as candidiasis, may occur and will add to the patient's discomfort.

Although the changes that affect the glands in the mucous membrane of the stomach are basically similar to the above, clinical findings are somewhat different, since the stomach is a more complicated structure that secretes enzymes (like pepsin) and hydrochloric acid in addition to mucus. A dose of about 1600 rads delivered in 10 days leads to diminution in all three secretions. This may be accompanied by nausea, and if the dose is substantially higher, hypoacidity becomes more pronounced. Hypoacidity, in addition to the accompanying changes of the mucous membrane, will add dyspepsia to the already existing symptoms. Subsequent pyloric spasm will complicate the picture further. Should the radiation insult continue, severe mucositis and ulceration results and leads to bleeding, hematemesis, and anemia. Radiation damage of such magnitude may prove sometimes to be fatal.

Further discussion concerning the changes affecting major salivary gland and other glands in the digestive system are deferred until later.

The *treatment* of mucous membrane radiation damage is both preventive and curative. Radiation must be conducted carefully and all normal tissues should be protected as adequately as possible. During the height of an inevitable reaction the mucous membrane should be given as much rest as possible, such as by no talking (involving laryngeal mucous membrane) and a light semisolid diet (involving the oral cavity and esophagus). Irritants like smoking, spicy food, excessive hot drinks, and liquor should be prohibited. Keeping the mucous membrane clean by rinsing or gargling is also helpful, in addition to combating secondary infection. It is imperative to try to diminish the dysfunction as much as possible; for example, a mixture of aspirin and glycerin (aspirin mucilage) may help deglutition. A close watch should be kept on the general condition of the patient to ensure that such functional changes do not reach an unacceptable level.

GLANDULAR TISSUES

Glands are found throughout the body and exist either in large discrete forms, like the parotid or thyroid glands, or in small glands embedded in various mucous membranes, like the mucous glands of the oral cavity or gastric glands of the stomach. The biological changes induced by irradiation to the latter have been described earlier. The glands that are most commonly exposed to irradiation are the major salivary, thyroid, and pituitary glands. The pancreas and suprarenal glands are exposed to irradiation to a much lesser degree.

Radiation damage to all glandular tissue is almost the same, varying only when certain physiological compensatory mechanisms exist, such as in the case with certain endocrine glands. The main damage caused by radiation can be summarized in three steps: (1) swelling and edema of the epithelia of the ducts, which may lead to their partial obstruction, followed by (2) damage to the acini, which results in the diminution of the secretion. (3) As radiation reaction heals, the damaged acini atrophy, with replacement by fibrous tissue, resulting in permanent reduction of the amount of secretion and loss of gland substance.

Major salivary glands

The major salivary glands are the parotid, submandibular (or submaxillary), and sublingual glands. The first is by far the largest and most important. Although all three secrete both serous and mucous fluids, the parotid is largely a serous gland. Radiation seems to affect serous acini more readily than it does mucous ones, leading to increased viscosity of the saliva, with such a change being noticed clinically after a dose of about 3000 rads in 3 weeks. A further radiation insult will lead to atrophy of a good proportion of the acini with more pronounced reduction in the quantity of secretions and increased acidity. As a result of these changes, the glands atrophy and lose substance (and weight). Healing of this radiation reaction is by fibrosis, which results in a small gland of a rather hard consistency. The only *treatment* available is protection of as much as possible of the bulk of the salivary gland during irradiation. Treatment of dryness of the mouth and difficulty in swallowing has been discussed earlier.

A secondary effect of the changes in the salivary secretion is damage to *teeth*. Teeth that are irradiated, or already unhealthy, are more liable to long-term changes and decay. Bad mouth hygiene contributes to this decay and hastens it. Some authors claim that extraction of such decayed teeth from an irradiated jaw may lead to massive necrosis, but recent experience with supervoltage and cobalt beams have shown that careful and well-timed extraction of teeth rarely had severe complications. Most of these teeth become loose because of resorption of the surrounding supporting structures, and their removal causes very little trauma, obviating in the most part the danger of massive necrosis. Prophylactic fluoride treatment during and after radiation diminishes damage to the tooth structure.

Thyroid gland

The thyroid gland is the largest endocrine gland often exposed to radiation damage by virtue of its proximity to tumors commonly treated by radiotherapy. Radiation to this gland can be delivered either by *external beams* or systemic radioactive isotopes (^{131}I). External irradiation leads to changes similar to those that afflict salivary glands (though at a higher dose level). Because of the relatively high radiation tolerance and the presence of compensatory mechanisms (such as hypertrophy of the remaining healthy acini), hypothyroidism is not a common complication. However, it may occur after a latent period of some months or years (such as after postmastectomy radiotherapy to the supraclavicular region). The best *treatment* is prophylactic by protection of the gland. Hormone replacement (thyroid extracts) in significant hypothyroidism is rarely necessary and often for a short period only. If radiation is delivered by systemic radioactive iodine (which is concentrated in the glandular acini), changes are usually more intense. The earliest reaction is radiation thyroiditis (tender, somewhat painful swelling of the gland) occurring a few days after the injection. It lasts a few days and usually subsides spontaneously. The subsequent damage to the thyroid acini results in diminished thyroid secretion. When the dose of ^{131}I is of the magnitude of 5 to 7 mc. (depending on the size of the gland), the damage may be only partial. That is why such a dose is used in the treatment of thyrotoxicosis, a condition characterized by increased metabolic activity. When the dose is of the magnitude of 80 to 100 mc. (depending on the size of the gland), the damage may be complete and lead to total ablation of the gland. In such a case almost all the acini become atrophic, with reduction in the mass of the gland and fibrous tissue replacement.

NERVOUS TISSUE

Very high doses of radiation lead to rapid death by its effect on the central nervous system. The following events have been reported in animal experiments: (1) ataxic phase (wherein the animal loses balance and ability of normal coordination of movement), (2) lethargic phase (wherein the animal becomes sluggish and lazy), (3) convulsive phase (wherein convulsions occur with increasing frequency until the animal passes into the terminal stage), (4) terminal phase followed by animal's death. The main cause of these events is a change in cellular permeability allowing greatly increased potassium levels in the blood.

However, such doses are almost never delivered during radiation therapy. Radiation damage resulting from doses used in radiotherapy is characterized by the presence of a latent period during which the organism displays no evidence of damage (both functionally and anatomically) followed by demonstrable damage. This damage is demonstrated histologically as areas of necrosis in the nervous tissue and is reflected clinically as a functional abnormality depending on the size and site of the necrotic area.

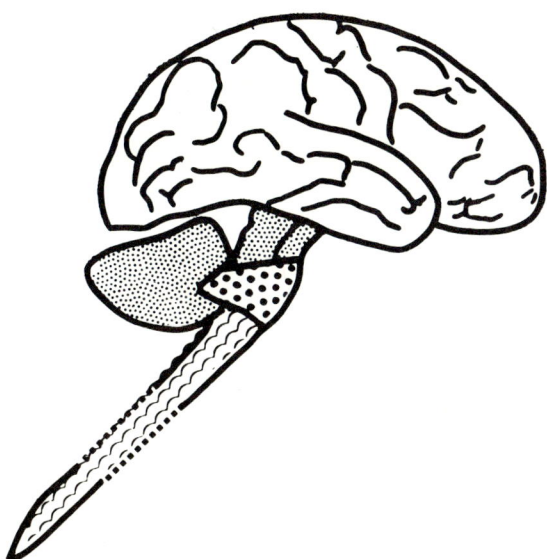

FIG. 5-1. Anatomy of central nervous system.

The response of the nervous tissue to radiation (delivered in therapeutic doses) depends on several factors, the most important of which are summarized as follows:

1. *Site irradiated.* The central nervous system varies in its tolerance to radiation. The midbrain including the medulla (see Fig. 5-1, anatomy of the CNS) and the spinal cord are the regions most vulnerable to radiation damage. The cerebral cortex and cerebellum seem to be more tolerant. It was also noticed that white matter is more prone to radiation damage than is gray matter. The peripheral nervous system is claimed to be most resistant to radiation damage. The spinal cord as a whole is noticeably vulnerable to radiation damage. Radiation myelopathy is characterized by three stages: First there is a relatively short latent period, and then there is early transient paresthesia (electric shocklike sensation occurring on flexion of the neck and radiating down the back and over the extremities—Lhermitte's syndrome), which may persist for some months. Ultimately it improves either spontaneously or gradually. This is followed by late irreversible myelopathy terminating in paresis or paralysis.

2. *Radiation dose/time and field size.* The higher the dose delivered to the nervous tissue and the shorter the time interval, the more likely is the possibility of radiation damage. This factor is directly linked to the volume of nervous tissue irradiated (or field size). It is estimated that a dose of 3650 to 4700 rads delivered in 3 weeks is biologically equivalent to 4500 to 5800 rads delivered to the same volume in 7 weeks.

3. *Maturation of tissue irradiated.* Immature mammalian neuroectodermal cells (called neuroblasts) found in the embryo are distinguished by their high vulnerability to radiation damage especially in the very early stages of development. These cells are usually killed by the process of cell reproductive death (see above). Such an incident may occur for instance if lengthy x-ray diagnostic procedures are carried out on pregnant women without due caution.

4. *Type of cell irradiated.* The central nervous system is composed of various types of cells with varying tolerance to radiation. These cells are the neuron, specialized neuronal receptors (rods and cones of the retina, olfactory neurons, taste neurons), and glial cells, which are the interstitial elements. It seems that the neuron is the cell most vulnerable to radiation damage. Transient changes may happen even after relatively small doses. The degree of damage depends on the part of the neuron receiving the brunt of radiation. The neuron is subdivided, according to anatomical and functional consideration (Fig. 5-2), into the perikaryon, dendrites, axons, and synapses. The perikaryon surrounds the nucleus and contains the major portion of metabolic machinery. From the perikaryon issue dendrites and the axon as the afferent and efferent conductive pathways of activity, respectively. The axon splits at its end into branches, each forming a presynaptic terminal. Each of these parts react differently to irradiation. It seems that relatively small doses of radiation may affect the function of the synapses even if histological (or anatomical) changes need a much higher

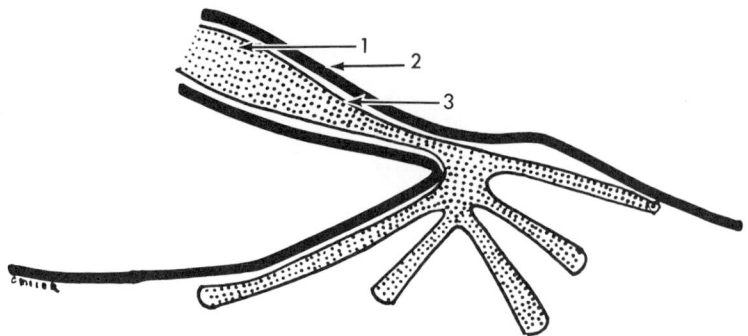

Fig. 5-2. Anatomy of neuron (axon and dendrites). 1, Axon. 2, Endoneurium (Schwann membrane). 3, Myelin sheath.

dose of radiation exposure to become demonstrable. The axon seems to be the most vulnerable part of the cell and reacts to the radiation injury by demyelination, that is, denudation of its myelin sheath. Myelin is a complex material consisting of sphingomyelin (lipidlike material and protein), which contains choline, an exquisitely radiosensitive material.

5. *Preexisting pathological conditions.* The existence of pathological conditions in the nervous tissue, such as a neoplastic process, increased intracranial tension or cerebrovascular disease, considerably decreases the tolerance of nervous tissue to radiation. The latent period in the presence of any of these conditions is noticeably reduced.

6. *Postirradiation factors.* The existence of certain pathological conditions, such as hypertension or hypothyroidism, in an organism in which the nervous tissue was irradiated may lead to shortening of the latent period or, in other words, enhance the radiation damage of the central nervous system. Even though the extent of damage to the central nerovus system by radiation is widely appreciated nowadays, *effective treatment* to the damage once it occurs hardly exists. Thus the best treatment is prophylaxis by protecting nervous tissue as much as possible and by the appreciation of the vital role of the time-dose relationship.

LYMPHOID, RETICULOENDOTHELIAL, AND HEMATOPOIETIC TISSUES

Lymphoid, reticuloendothelial, and hematopoietic tissues not only display a common notable radiosensitivity, but they are also related morphologically. Some authors have claimed that the parent cells of the hematopoietic tissues (the stem cell) are the small lymphocytes of the bone marrow. However, our discussion is conducted under two separate headings: effect on hematopoietic tissues and effect on lymphoreticular tissues and lymphocytes.

Effect on hematopoietic tissues

For a proper understanding of the effect of radiation on hematopoietic tissues their anatomy as well as their function must be clarified as shown in Table 5-1. Hematopoietic tissues are divided into two components: *blood-forming tissues* and *circulating blood elements*. The former are found mainly in the bone marrow (called active marrow) and rarely in the liver, whereas the latter are found in the peripheral blood. Active marrow is found mainly in flat bones in adults (especially the pelvis) and metaphyses of long bones. The shaft of long bones may contain active marrow in children and in times of stress, otherwise it is a fatty inactive element. The marrow contains the parent cell as well as the dividing and differentiating stages of

TABLE 5-1. Hematopoietic tissues

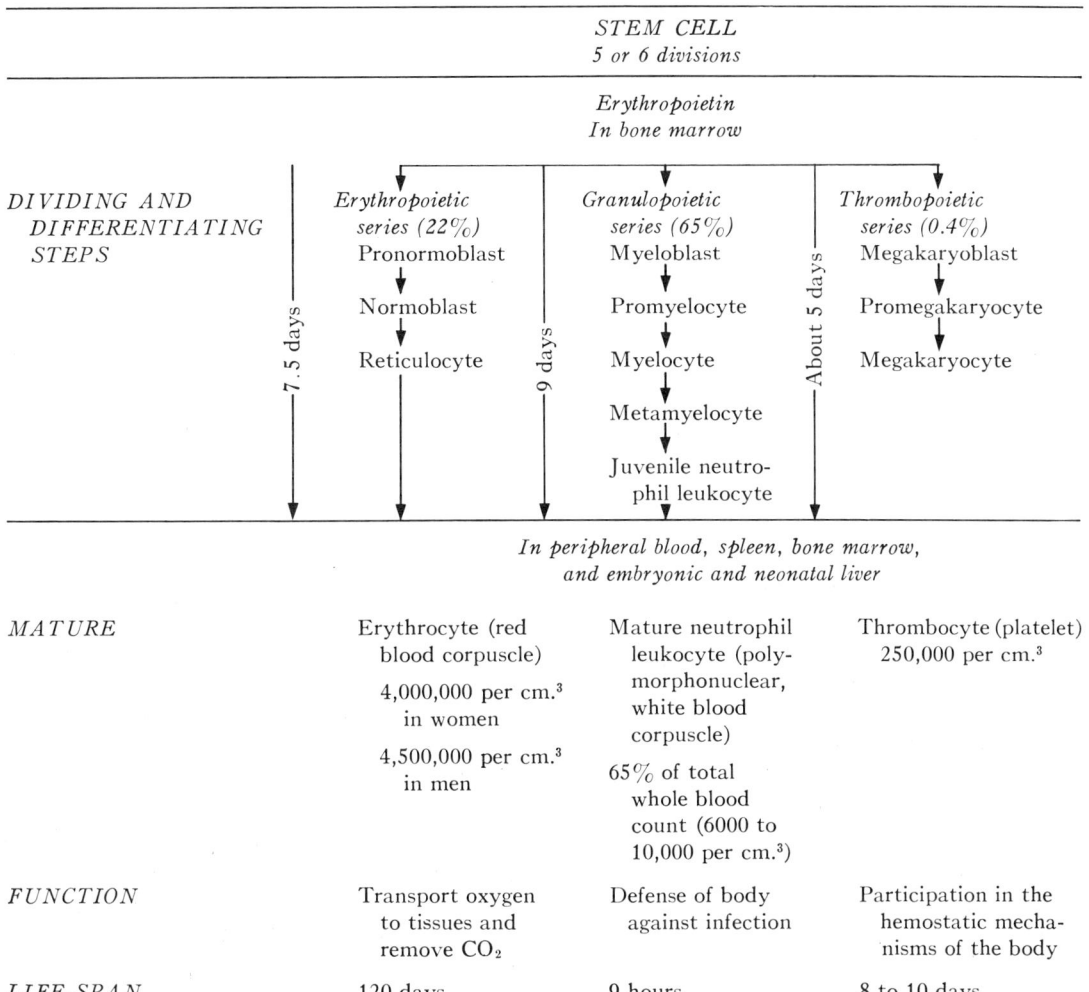

the erythropoietic, granulopoietic, and thrombopoietic elements. The peripheral blood contains the mature forms of these elements. However, less mature forms may escape to the peripheral blood in times of stress (such as inflammations and leukemias).

Effect of radiation on blood-forming tissues. The effect of radiation on the blood-forming tissues (especially the stem cell) depends on various factors: physical, target, and environmental. The *physical factors* are summarized as follows:

1. *Dose fractionation.* A large single dose has an effect different from the same dose divided among several fractions.

2. *Continuous irradiation.* Continuous irradiation over a protracted period seems to have a more deleterious effect than does the same dose given in one fraction (to the stem cell).

3. *Field size and site.* The effect of irradiating larger volumes of bone (and bone marrow) is quite profound. This is more so if the volume includes a large amount of active marrow (pelvis or spine) as compared to areas

where the bone marrow is dormant or fatty (shafts of long bones).
4. *Characteristics of the beam.* Particle beams such as neutrons possess a higher relative biological efficiency (RBE, see glossary) than does a ^{60}Co beam.

Target factors mean the effect of radiation (in comparable physical factors) on various components of the bone marrow. The *stem cell* (or parent cell) displays the following changes:
1. *Loss of reproductive capacity.* This may be estimated by using the standard of LD_{50} per 30 days (see glossary), whereby death occurs in experimental animals after total body irradiation because of the failure of bone marrow. This results from inability of the stem cell to repopulate the bone marrow and peripheral blood after the degeneration of the blood elements by natural means or irradiation.
2. *Lethal effect (or death).* Death of the stem cell is usually assessed by use of the D_0 value (see glossary).

Erythropoietic tissue is quite vulnerable to radiation damage, particularly the early cells in the development series. However, it recovers fairly quickly. It is more affected by acute large doses than by repeated small doses (chronic irradiation). *Granulopoietic tissue* is next in vulnerability but with the difference that "chronic" irradiation has a relatively more profound effect. The *thrombopoietic series* seems also to be quite vulnerable and somewhat slow to recover. As a result of all these changes, the *bone marrow* becomes depleted of its cells in addition to the damage to the marrow architecture itself. However, all these changes are reversible, with a rate depending on the dose given, the amount, and the site of marrow affected.

Environmental factors play an important role in modifying radiation damage. The two most important are the effect of hypoxia (an oxygen enhancement ratio [see glossary] of over 2 was measured in some experiments) and the presence of chemical protectors (such as cystamine, which has a rather temporary protective effect).

Effect of radiation on circulating blood elements. Circulating blood elements (red blood corpuscles, white blood corpuscles, and platelets) have a limited natural life-span (Table 5-1), after which they degenerate while their number is replenished from the blood-forming organs. Thus a change in their number after irradiation of a large section of the body may be caused by damage of both the blood-forming tissues as well as the circulating elements themselves. In the following paragraphs, we have summarized the most important facts about the changes affecting the blood elements after irradiation:

Red blood corpuscles (erythrocytes). (1) Their number may be reduced as a result of loss through hemorrhages and injury to vessel walls (caused by radiation). (2) Radiation has an indirect life-shortening effect. (3) Younger cells may be able to stand radiation insult better than older ones can.

Granulocytes (polymorphonuclear white blood corpuscles). At the beginning of irradiation there is a decrease in the cell count (dose dependent), followed by an abortive rise, but ultimately the numbers continue to decrease persistently.

Platelets (thrombocytes). Platelets are rather resistant cells, and the decrease in their number noticed with radiation is attributable to the effect on the blood-forming organs. The result of radiation is thrombocytopenia (dose dependent), which will ultimately affect the clotting mechanism of the blood by impeding the following functions: formation of platelet plugs, interaction of platelets and serum clotting factors, platelet-related vasoconstrictor substance, and clot retraction.

The *clinical manifestations* of damage to the hematopoietic tissues are numerous and include anemia, neutropenia (reduction in the number of circulating white cells), and thrombocytopenia. Aplasia of the bone marrow may occur in extreme cases.

Treatment should be aggressive to prevent inevitable complications. Blood transfusion, iron medications, and antibiotics are the mainstay of treatment. In severe cases of neutropenia the patient may have to be isolated as a protection against infections (even the simplest infection may prove fatal).

Transfusions with bone marrow cells have been used in some cases (especially in accidents involving nuclear reactors) with a certain degree of success, but the process is technically difficult and too early to evaluate properly. It will be discussed in more detail later on.

Effect on lymphoreticular tissues and lymphocytes

The parent cells are found in lymph nodes, lymphoid organs (spleen, tonsils, thymus), and bone marrow. The mature cells are found in the peripheral blood and form about 25% of the total white blood cells. The functions of the lymphocytes are not clearly defined but they are claimed to include the following:

1. They form the hematopoietic stem cell, which has been discussed previously.
2. They participate in the immune mechanism.
3. They are claimed to give their DNA to other proliferating cells, such as regenerating liver cells.

The effect of radiation on lymphoreticular tissue (lymph nodes and spleen), lymphocytes, and other such parts is now discussed.

The construction of a typical *lymph node* is seen in Fig. 5-3. It is composed of lymphocytes and lymphoblasts, which are supported by a fibrous framework containing the blood vessels. Lymph passes into the node through lymph sinuses and then between the lymphocytes, phagocytic reticulum cells, and macrophages. It is then collected by an efferent system. Each of these elements (lymphocytes, fibrous framework, and macrophages) exhibits different radiosensitivities. *Lymphocytes,* especially the small type, are highly vulnerable to radiation damage, and the nodes may be almost completely denuded within a few hours after a high dose of irradiation. These changes are dose dependent. The *macrophages on reticuloendothelial elements* are

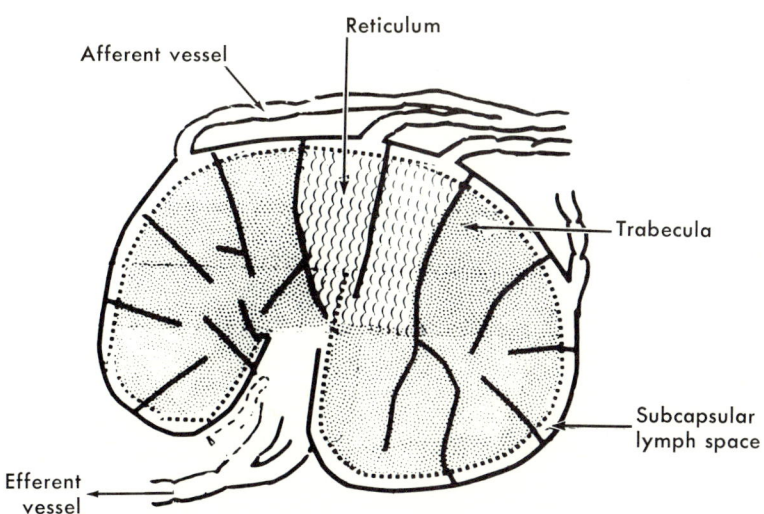

Fig. 5-3. Scheme of lymph node.

somewhat less vulnerable, but a relatively high dose may lead to decrease in their physiological activities. The *fibrous framework* seems to be more vulnerable to chronic irradiation with gradual increase in the connective tissue, leading to complete disruption of the normal architecture of the lymph node structure. *Lymphatic vessels* seem to be relatively radioresistant and are disrupted only because of radiation-induced increase in fibrous tissue, which may impair their potency.

The *spleen* is very similar to lymph nodes both in structure and radiosensitivity. It is composed of white pulp (rich in lymphocytes) and red pulp (rich in phagocytic reticulum cells in a fibrous framework). The white pulp is the most sensitive to radiation insult, which may lead to the total depletion of lymphocytes. The elements of the red pulp are more resistant. As a sequence of radiation changes, the spleen shrinks rapidly to only a part of its normal weight. This occurs whether radiation is delivered directly to the spleen or to other lymphatic tissue (lymphocyte pool), a phenomenon termed the "abscopal effect" (see glossary). Regeneration and recovery is claimed to occur after the conversion of reticular cells to lymphoblasts and gradually increasing lymphopoiesis. Radiation also alters the physiologic functions of the spleen, which are its ability to store red blood cells, its erythrolytic (ability to destroy red blood cells) activity, capacity for storing iron pigments, and production of antibodies.

EFFECT OF RADIATION ON IMMUNITY

Immunity, which represents the body's defense mechanism, is dependent on an intact lymphoreticulo-hemopoietic system; for example, the initial antibody response of an acquired immunity is apparently dependent on a process that requires intact lymphoctyes and plasma cells. This was predicted by Murphy as early as 1914. Later experimentation showed that whole body irradiation depresses both the innate and acquired immunity by its effect on the lymphoreticular system. Protection of the lymphocyte pool (spleen, appendix, lymph nodes, and others) will reduce the degree of immunosuppression after irradiation.

The degree of immune response suppression is dependent on several factors, some of which are summarized as follows:

1. Dose-time characteristics. High dose rates (100 R per minute or greater) has more profound effect than low dose rates (10 R per minute or less).
2. Timing of the irradiation in relation to the immunological process. Irradiation 1 or 2 days before antigen introduction causes significant delay and reduction in peak antibody titer. On the other hand, irradiation delivered 2 hours after antigen introduction delays the appearance of antibody, but the peak titer is higher than in nonirradiation control. Irradiation delivered 2 days after antigen introduction seems to result only in the delay of the appearance of antibody.
3. Route of administration of the antigenic stimulus.
4. Type of immunological process involved, that is, cellular versus antigen antibody. It is claimed that cellular (or cell-mediated) immune response becomes greater after local irradiation. This may be explained by the accelerated proliferation of competent cells surviving radiation damage. The clinical application of this is noticed in the beneficial effect of small doses of radiation delivered to some inflammatory lesions. However, such an approach is rarely used nowadays and is largely historical.

The effect of radiation on immunity to cancer is still a largely speculative field. Although irradiation may affect immunity adversely, it seems that irradiating large tumors as well as grossly diseased lymph nodes successfully may help to improve the immunological status of the patient.

LEUKEMOGONIC EFFECTS OF RADIATION

It is now accepted that radiation may be the cause of leukemia in man. Three sources of information lead to this conclusion:

1. Data from the survivors of the atomic bomb in Hiroshima and Nagasaki show that granulocytic leukemia in its acute form predominated.
2. Patients with benign diseases (usually ankylosing spondylitis) and long-life expectancy given substantial therapeutic irradiation died from subsequent leukemia at a rate 5 to 10 times higher than the rate in a comparable normal nonradiated group.
3. Early workers in radiology (physicists, physicians, and technicians) died sooner than normal. The deaths from leukemia in radiologists in the period 1928 to 1948 was nine times that in other physicians in the same period. However, this incidence dropped to about half (4 to 5 times) in the period 1949 to 1958, probably because of improved radiation protection.

Radiation-induced leukemia was found to have the following characteristics: (1) A latent period is rather long (maybe as long as 12 years). In the atomic-bomb survivors, the peak was observed 5 to 8 years after the explosion. (2) The type of leukemia noticed appears to be the acute form with some cases of chronic granulocytic leukemia. (3) There does not seem to be a threshold dose although those closest to the bomb's hypocenter had a relatively high incidence of leukemia. (4) A linear dose-response relationship seems to exist. A single large exposure (as occurred with the atomic bomb) produced a greater incidence of leukemia than the same dose given over a period of years. (5) Susceptibility to leukemia seems to decrease with increasing age of the individual. Therefore newborns and infants seem to be more susceptible.

KIDNEYS

The kidneys are probably the most radiosensitive organs in the abdomen. The pathological changes of radiation damage depend largely on the dose delivered. The clinical picture depends on the dose delivered to the volume of kidney tissue irradiated. Generally these changes are classified into two forms—acute and chronic.

Acute radiation damage. The earliest changes noticed are in the laboratory tests —diminished renal plasma flow, glomerular filtration rate, and tubular excretory capacity, which may occur after doses as small as 400 rads. With higher doses the renal blood flow shows a transient increase followed by an eventual and steady decrease. Histological examination of the kidneys during this period reveals no striking changes. Clinically the earliest findings will be proteinuria.

If the radiation dose to a substantial amount of renal tissue is high, hypertension, anemia, and cardiomegaly may predominate and the kidney becomes atrophic and fibrotic. Both the tubules and glomeruli are affected and give rise to a picture of acute glomerulonephritis. The fate of the patients affected in this fashion varies, but almost all of them are left with a degree of chronic nephritis. About one third of these patients suffer from progressively increasing hypertension (malignant hypertension), which is invariably fatal. Another group may die of renal failure some years later. Treatment would depend on hypotensive drugs, renal care, and probably renal dialysis. When only one kidney is damaged (leading to malignant hypertension), nephrectomy may be curative.

Chronic changes. Chronic changes may either follow an earlier acute radiation nephritis or start anew. The latter is more common and occurs in about 40% of the cases where a dose of 2500 to 3250 rads was delivered in 3 to 6 weeks to both kidneys. There is a lag period of varying lengths (up to 8 years in some cases) between the irradiation and incidence of the syndrome during which the individual's renovascular functions are apparently within normal. The usual clinical picture is that of hypertension, anemia, weakness, proteinurea, urinary casts, and raised blood urea. The severity of the syndrome depends not only on the dose time delivered but also on the proportion of renal tissue irradiated. Histologically the kidney displays a picture of vascular damage, tubular atrophy, glomerular hyalinization, and interstitial fibrosis. The treatment is the same as in chronic glomerulonephritis attributable to other causes—hypotensive drugs, renal care, and dialysis.

Because of the danger of radiation nephritis, the following steps must be taken whenever radiation is employed to treat an organ near the kidneys: (1) complete protection of both kidneys if possible, (2) protection of as much renal tissue as possible if the inclusion of some renal tissue in the treated volume is inevitable, and (3) whenever possible a limitation of the dose delivered to renal tissue to less than 2000 rads in 2 weeks or its biological equivalent.

LUNGS

Fig. 5-4 shows a schematic representation of the lower air passages composed of the bronchial tree and alveoli. The epithelial lining changes from columnar ciliated in the former to flat in the latter. Radiation damage to the lungs, the so-called radiation pneumonitis, is essentially caused by changes in the alveolar wall coupled with accumulation of exudate in the air sac. Radiation damage to the trachea and larger bronchi is essentially that of the mucous membrane (discussed earlier).

Radiation pneumonitis may be divided into three phases:

1. The *earliest changes* are hyperemia (congestion) and increased transudate accompanied with degeneration of lymph follicles. This may be reflected clinically as cough productive of sputum. This occurs in the first few days of treatment especially if the initial doses are high. Radiological examination of the chest at this stage shows no departure from normal.

2. The *degenerative stage* occurs when the dose is high or given in a short time. In its full-blown picture the changes are swelling and later sloughing of the alveolar cells, conspicuous edema, and a hyaline membrane continuous with the fibrous tissue of the alveolar wall. The pleura is thickened with the presence of fibropurulent pleuritis. Such a picture is probably fatal and should never occur with therapeutic regimens although it may occur at the end of a radical course of treatment (or up to 8 weeks later) where there is a preexisting lung pathological condition (such as infection). The cough continues to increase and sputum may become thick and white. Increasing degrees of dyspnea are evident, in addition to often spiking fever and night sweats. Radiological ex-

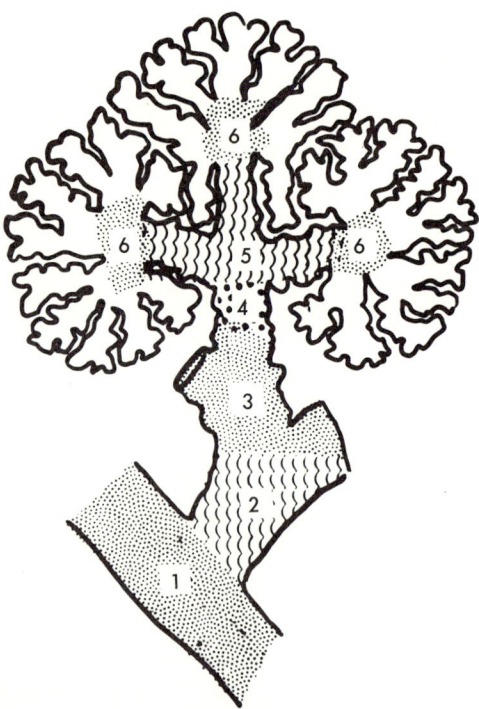

FIG. 5-4. Diagram showing bronchioles, terminal bronchioles, and air sacs. **1**, Terminal bronchiole. **2 and 3**, Respiratory bronchioles. **4**, Terminal respiratory bronchiole. **5**, Alveolar ducts. **6**, Atrium leading to air saccules.

amination may show signs of atelectasis, increased clouding of the lungs, or signs of pleural reaction. However, in the presence of a preexisting lung pathological condition, these changes may be concealed, overlooked, or too difficult to interpret. The treatment would depend on the particulars of a certain case, but suspension of radiation (or modification of the plan of treatment), appropriate antibiotics, steroid medication, and inhalation therapy are the main methods to be considered.

The full-blown picture described above is rarely encountered in radiation therapy. Instead, after a dose of about 4500 rads given in about 4 weeks, patients may complain of increasing cough, dyspnea, and fever. X-ray films may show a mixture of any of the above-described findings. Patients usually respond well to antibiotics, which may be combined with steroids in certain cases.

3. The *regenerative stage* is manifested by proliferation of the connective tissue in the lung parenchyma leading to different fibrotic changes. Proliferation of bronchial epithelia may also occur in addition to fibrotic changes (and thickening of the pleura). If lung destruction (in the degenerative phase) was extensive, permanent extensive fibrosis may ensue. Complications like multiple abscesses may occur. The clinical picture is that of cough as well as hemoptysis, dyspnea, and orthopnea. Clubbing of fingers and other cyanotic phenomena may also occur. Signs and symptoms related to complications (such as abscess) may also exist. Radiological findings will depend on the pathological changes in each case, but atelectasis, opacities, pleural thickening, and mediastinal and hilar abnormalities are very common. The clinical and roentgenographic picture of radiation pneumonitis may closely simulate that of the primary tumor. Treatment of this stage of radiation pneumonitis is similar to that in stage 2, but still prophylaxis by careful planning and execution of treatment is the best method of management.

Radiological changes in the chest and radiation pneumonitis

It is worthwhile mentioning that there is no direct relationship between radiological changes and the degree of clinical damage. Very often the x-ray films demonstrate large areas of opacities, for instance, in the apex after the treatment of supraclavicular fields while the patient is absolutely free of symptoms and clinical signs. This is partly because of the presence of reserve capacity in the lungs, hypertrophy of the remaining lung tissues, and other compensatory physiological mechanisms. Obviously such cases need no active treatment.

CHAPTER 6

EFFECT OF RADIATION ON THE WHOLE BODY

Radiation may affect the whole body, depending on whether it is delivered in a relatively short time (whether as a single dose, such as an accidental exposure in an atomic plant, or as regular doses in a few weeks), leading to what may be called an acute radiation effect, or in a relatively very long time (such as from natural sources or as atomic fallout), leading to what may be termed "chronic radiation effect."

CHRONIC RADIATION EFFECT

This results from long-term irradiation over many years. The sources of such radiation are either natural or man made. Natural sources are cosmic radiation, terrestrial radiation, and radiation from thorium, uranium, and radium in soil and produce an estimated mean total yearly dose of 0.1 rem (see glossary). Man-made sources include medical irradiation (diagnostic x-ray procedures and radiation therapy) and fallout from atomic-weapon tests. Fallout affects man by two methods—externally by air contamination to a minimal degree and internally by the ingestion of fission products, mainly strontium (^{90}Sr) and to a much lesser degree calcium. The biological cycle of these products is seen in Fig. 6-1.

The possible biological effects of these radiations are genetic, leukemia induction, and other delayed effects. The genetic effect of radiation on humans can only be deduced from animal experiments. Although such deductions may not be accurate, they are still logical, since there is no cause to suggest that *Homo sapiens* (man) is totally different from other animal species. The mutagenic effect of radiation is well established and has been discussed earlier. The induction of leukemia was discussed earlier in detail.

Among the most significant delayed effects is life shortening from increased incidence of malignant disease. Researchers found that there is an increased mortality from skin cancer, pancreatic cancer, and leukemia among medical men who entered radiological practice before 1921.

It is reasonable to conclude that ionizing radiation from any source represents a hazard that should be weighed very carefully to obviate its indiscriminate use. The recent developments of the partial ban on atomic

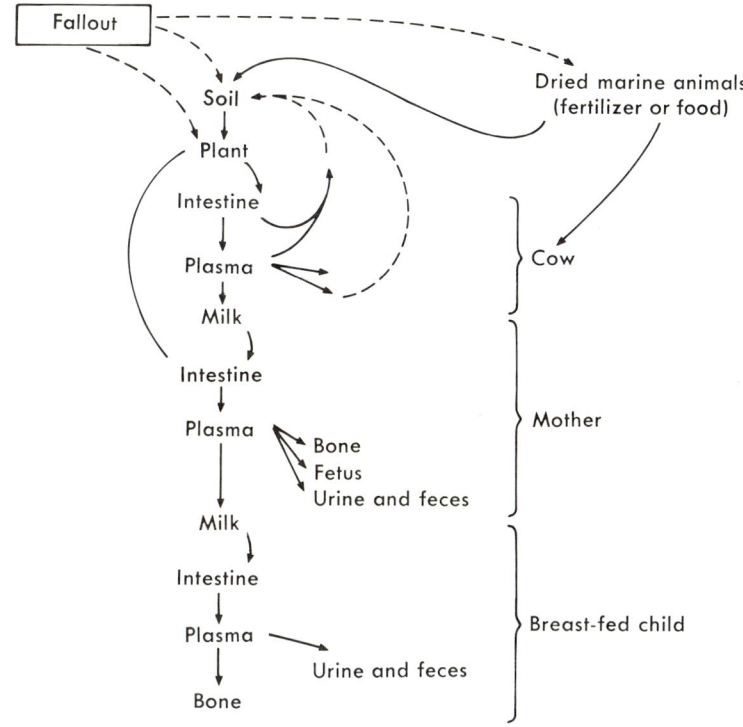

Fig. 6-1. Biological cycle of calcium and strontium 90. (Redrawn from Bacq, Z. M., and Alexander, P.: Fundamentals of radiobiology, London, 1961, Pergamon Press.)

testing is no doubt a step in the right direction.

ACUTE EFFECT OF RADIATION

Radiation sickness has two causes. The most common is therapeutic radiation (given to a large volume of tissues); the second (and much more rare) is whole-body exposure to radiation and may be either therapeutic (during the treatment of some forms of leukemia or childhood sarcomas, such as Ewing's sarcoma) or accidental from exposure to high dose radiations in some nuclear plants (as happened in Yugoslavia where six young scientists were accidentally irradiated at Vinča or in the U.S.A. where five men were affected at the Y-12 plan) or the experience of Hiroshima and Nagasaki. Although radiation sickness from either large volumes of radiation therapy or whole-body exposure may be basically similar, it differs so much in magnitude that they should be considered separately.

Whole-body irradiation

Radiation sickness from whole-body irradiation is totally dose dependent. The LD_{50} (see glossary) is probably around 700 roentgens (R) for young adults. A rem is defined as the absorbed dose in rads multiplied by the relative biological efficiency (RBE, see glossary). Total body exposure to 850 R is probably fatal if not treated promptly.

The *clinical picture* of acute radiation sickness depends mainly on the dose given, but the age of the individual and his state of health may also play a minor role. Young adults are a better risk than children or elderly people. Symptoms usually occur after a latent period of variable length, depending on the exposure dose, with an average of 2 weeks. A low dose (100 to 200 rems) causes mild nausea, vomiting, and mental depression. If the dose is much smaller than 100 rems, symptoms may be absent. When the dose is around 200 rems, symptoms may be of such magnitude that they may necessitate some treatment. Vomiting particularly is an extremely regular symptom, so much so that its severity may be used to estimate the dose of exposure if this is not known accurately. It is probably of central nervous system origin. Symptoms are best treated by antiemetics, such as prochlorperazine dimaleate (Compazine), in addition to general maintenance measures (rest, diet, and vitamins).

High dose. Vomiting becomes persistent and may be accompanied by diarrhea. Diarrhea implies a bad prognosis, especially if it occurs early after exposure. Epilation of hair becomes noticed after about 2 weeks. This is followed by depression of the *hematopoietic system,* which is evidenced by diminution in almost all the blood constituents, which are the white cells, lymphocytes, platelets, and red blood corpuscles. Abnormal blood components appear (such as bilobed lymphocytes) and other normal indicators disappear (such as reticulocytes, indicating absence of red cell regeneration). There may result hemorrhages, which are probably related to platelet deficiency, since it can be checked by platelet transfusions.

Mental depression becomes evident and may sometimes take serious dimensions. Ulcerations of *mucous membranes,* such as oropharyngeal or intestinal wall, compound the gastrointestinal symptoms of colic, vomiting, and diarrhea. This will eventually lead to *water and electrolyte imbalance.*

Spermatozoa count is quite a sensitive indicator, and temporary disappearance is a very regular observation when the dose has reached 400 rem. Apparently *ovaries* are more resistant to radiation effect than are the *testes.*

Polyurea may also occur but there is little change in total urinary nitrogen.

The *immune mechanism* of the body is depressed, a condition that would make infections more dangerous and widespread.

Complications may arise at any time. The most common are infection, hemorrhage, and shock. These were particularly serious in the Hiroshima and Nagasaki aftereffects as compared to accidental exposures. Whether this is related to the race of the individuals, their previous state of health, or availability of adequate treatment measures is still debatable.

Treatment. The most important treatment measures are hospital rest, attention to general care (adequate diet and fluid), and treatment of complications especially the hemorrhage and anemia. Anemia is particularly important if exposure is above 500 rems where hematologic death is the most common complication. This is best treated by bone marrow transplantation or transfusion. About 300 to 400 cc. are obtained from an appropriate donor by several bone aspirations (under general anesthesia) and injected intravenously. This method can be lifesaving. The higher the exposure dose, the earlier should be the time of institution of the transplant.

Radiation sickness from large-volume radiation therapy

This is the type most commonly encountered by the radiation therapist and still rather vague in etiology. It is not always dependent on volume, dose, type of tumor, or general condition of the patient. However, it is encountered more often where a large volume, including abdominal organs and especially the liver, is being treated. It starts a few days after the beginning of a radiation therapy course, usually the second or third week and lasts for about 1 or 2 weeks. Women are more susceptible to it than are men. It is characterized by nausea and vomiting and sometimes a feeling of malaise. The patient's appetite may be affected, leading to weight loss and feeling of weakness and ill-being, especially if proper attention to calorie intake and proper diet is lacking.

The symptoms are usually mild and rarely necessitate active measures. However, if the general condition of the patient, weight, and nutrition, suffer then antiemetics are helpful. Reassurance and kind understanding by the doctor-technician axis are usually more effective than any one drug. Studies have shown that this phenomenon tends to occur more in general wards that contain a large population of patients receiving radiation therapy. Such findings indicate the presence of a strong psychological element, and some trials that compared an antiemetic and a placebo seemed to confirm this psychological element. The effect of radiation therapy given during the treatment of malignancies on various body systems would depend on the site of the treated volume and has been discussed earlier in this chapter.

CHAPTER 7

EFFECT OF RADIATION ON MALIGNANT TUMORS

The premise upon which radiation therapy of malignant tumors hinges is the difference in vulnerability (a sensitivity) to radiation damage between malignant cells and normal ones. The main cause of such a difference is the fact that tumor cells are more active and less differentiated. We have already shown that such conditions are prerequisites for radiation-induced cell damage. The *therapeutic ratio* is the difference between the radiation dose necessary to destroy a malignant cell or a group of cells (a tumor) (called the *tumor lethal dose*) and that which would inflict the same degree of injury on the surrounding normal tissue (called *tissue tolerance*). Obviously the larger this difference (or ratio), the higher is the sensitivity of this tumor to radiation (or its radiosensitivity). The higher the radiosensitivity of a tumor, the more is the likelihood of control of local disease by radiation. Since this is an important end to which all radiotherapy is directed, it is essential to study the factors that affect radiosensitivity. Most of these factors are the result of clinical observation; some are confirmed by radiobiological experiments, but nearly all are still only partially understood. The most significant of these factors are summarized as follows.

Oxygen tension. Experiments have shown that the higher the oxygen tension (of a cell) the higher the radiosensitivity (Fig. 7-1). This also holds in clinical observation as necrotic tumors with poor blood supply (and low oxygen tension) are rather radioresistant. As a result, the technique of irradiating patients under high oxygen tension (hyperbaric oxygen chambers) evolved. Its results and indication are still controversial.

The reverse of the above finding is also true, hypoxic cells (with lower oxygen tension) are less radiosensitive. As the physiological response of normal tissues to generalized hypoxia is more pronounced than that of malignant ones (which become relatively more oxygenated), it follows that the effect of radiation therapy under hypoxia will be more noticeable on malignant

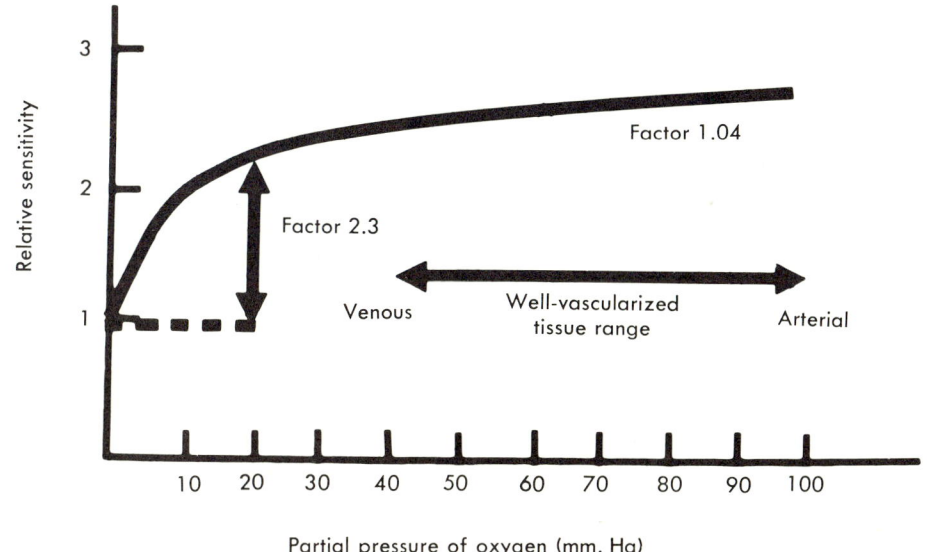

Fig. 7-1. Variation in relative radiosensitivity with variation in tension of dissolved oxygen. (Redrawn from Gary, L. H.: Brit. J. Radiol. 30:403, 1957.)

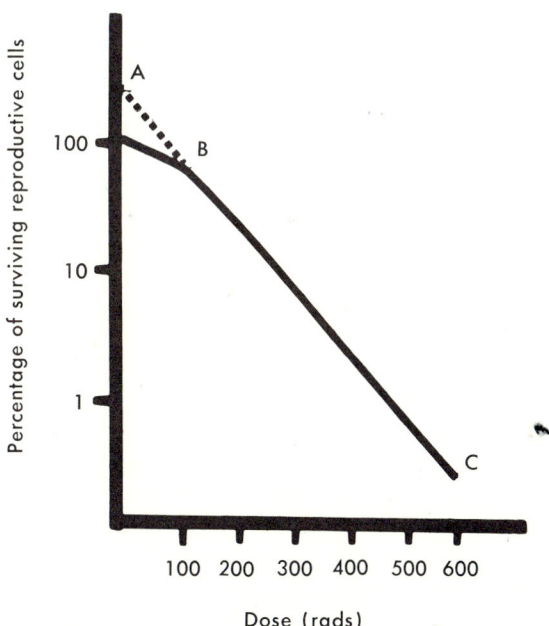

Fig. 7-2. Typical cell-survival curve, showing the proportion of surviving cells with reproductive capacity after a given dose. Note the shoulder of the curve, indicating minimal (sublethal) damage. The straight-line portion (slope) shows increased (lethal) damage or death.

cells. However, hypoxia has other serious effects on the body systems so that such a technique has not been widely used.

Fractionation. A dose of radiation given to a cell population inflicts a certain degree of damage (to their reproductive integrity), as expressed in Fig. 7-2, which indicates that below a certain dosage the damage is sublethal, after which point it increases progressively, ultimately causing cell death. If several small doses are given successively, the result is a certain degree of cellular recovery, or *repair,* during the periods between the successive doses, as represented in Fig. 7-3. Although a maximum effect may be obtained if a single large dose is delivered rather than the same dose given as several small fractions, normal tissues will be damaged in such a way that the therapeutic ratio of this regimen is too low to be beneficial. Therapists also found that recovery of normal tissues (during the periods between successive doses) is more appreciable than that of malignant tissues. Moreover fractionated doses lead to successive reduction of the tumor size through

76 *Biological effects of radiation*

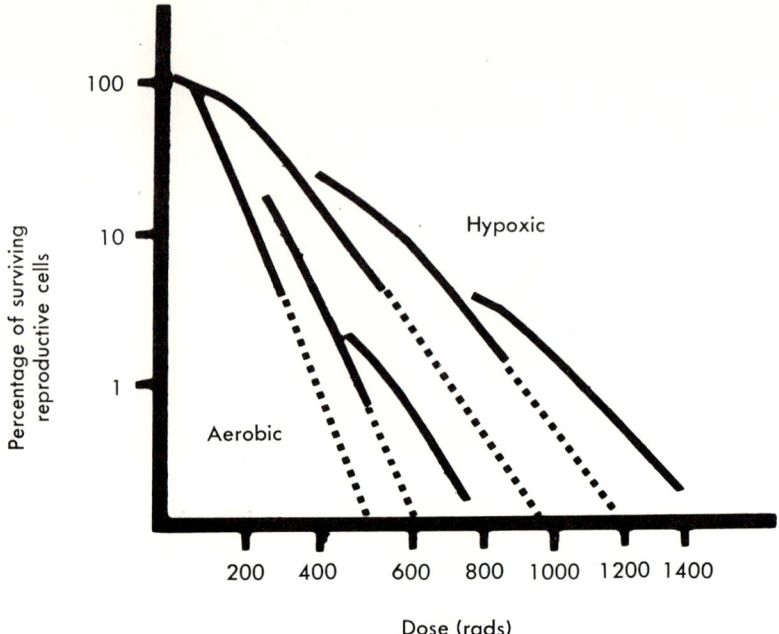

Fig. 7-3. Comparison of results of fractionated irradiation of a cell culture during aerobic and hypoxic states. (Redrawn from Moss, W. T., and Brand, W. N.: Therapeutic radiology, St. Louis, 1969, The C. V. Mosby Co.)

destruction of the well-oxygenated radiosensitive portion. Since the blood supply of the tumor continues to be fairly constant, that of the residuum is then relatively increased. The result is an improved oxygen tension (with the assumption that the oxygen tension of a tumor remains constant during irradiation) rendering the residuum more radiosensitive. Moreover, the blood vessels that had been compressed by the tumor are decompressed as it shrinks by successive fractions, leading to better oxygenation and improved radiosensitivity. The number of fractions and the time length between them, expressed in practical radiotherapy as the dose-time relation, is one of the most important (and still not fully understood) concepts in radiotherapy. The optimal number of fractions has not been determined yet, and the different systems in use have been chosen empirically. However, certain rules should guide the radiotherapist in deciding about the number of fractions. These are summarized as follows: (1) The greater the mitotic activity of a certain tumor, the shorter should be the interval between fractions (to avoid a high percentage of tumor recovery); (2) the longer the interval between fractions, the lesser is the damage to normal cells (important for normal tissues, known for their radiosensitivity); (3) the greater the dose of each fraction, the greater the biological effect.

Volume irradiated. The relation between tissue tolerance and the volume irradiated is an important established premise in radiotherapy. The larger the volume irradiated, the less is the tissue tolerance. Thus, the larger the volume irradiated, the less is the therapeutic ratio. Moreover, a large irradiated volume would mean a larger tumor. The larger cancer not only has more cells (necessitating a larger dose and meaning a correspondingly lower therapeutic ratio), but the cells are generally less sensi-

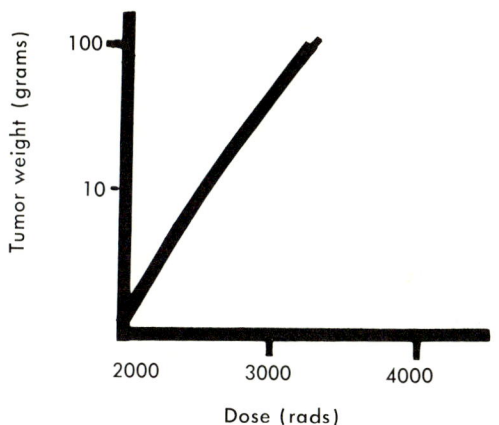

Fig. 7-4. Relationship of the size of a cancer to the single dose necessary for cure.

tive because of relatively poor oxygenation (Fig. 7-4).

Tumor cell type. The cell type is an important aspect upon which radiosensitivity is dependent. As a rule squamous cell carcinomas and adenocarcinomas are more sensitive than are connective tissue sarcomas. Tumors of lymphoreticular origin display the highest radiosensitivity.

Site of a tumor. The site of a tumor, or the tumor bed, obviously plays a most important role in deciding radiosensitivity since it is the other half of the therapeutic ratio. This effect may be attributable to several factors: a site with a better blood supply affords a better blood supply to the tumor and thus improves its radiosensitivity. Certain sites, such as the perineum, are known by their poor toleranec to radiation whereas others, such as the uterine cervix are known by their high tolerance.

Phase of cell cycle. Researchers noticed experimentally that cellular radiosensitivity is maximal just before the phase of DNA synthesis and minimal during the phase itself. Presumably if all the cells in a malignant tumor are in the same phase, it would be feasible to try to deliver radiation during the proper moment, but this assumption does not exist in clinical practice where the cells of any tumor are in varying degrees of division (or activity) or are altogether dormant.

SECTION THREE

CLINICAL RADIATION ONCOLOGY

In this section we will deal with clinical oncology from the radiotherapist's point of view or, in other words, the place of radiation therapy in the treatment of malignant diseases in different systems. As the role of radiotherapy varies from one system to the other and from one tumor to the other, stress will be placed on areas where radiation therapy plays a major role. While it is customary to discuss malignant tumors according to their anatomical system or site of origin, one must remember that very often cancer does not respect the usual anatomical boundaries. Sometimes it is virtually impossible to identify the site of origin of a lesion, such as tumors of upper air and food passages. Yet the site and the tissue of origin very often decide a tumor's behavior and response to radiation. For that reason malignant lesions will be discussed according to their site of origin.

CHAPTER 8

INTRODUCTION TO NEOPLASIA

The word "neoplasia," which literally means 'new' *(neo-)* 'growth' or 'form' (*plassein,* 'to form') has been chosen instead of the word "cancer" to introduce the reader to the various problems of malignant diseases, since the term "cancer" is rather controversial in its definition. Neoplasms are conventionally classified into benign and malignant. The delineating line separating the two is sometimes vague and often a neoplasm that started as a benign lesion changes its character to become malignant.

Neoplasms are broadly classified into epithelial, endothelial, or mesothelial according to the cell of origin. Malignant tumors of epithelial origin are called carcinomas, those from mesothelial or endothelial origins are generally termed sarcomas. The terminology of benign tumors has tended to derive from the tissue of origin; for example, bones have osteoma, fatty tissues have lipoma, muscle tissues have myoma, fibrous tissues have fibroma, and so on. For the rest of this chapter the most outstanding characteristics of benign and malignant neoplasms are compared and discussed.

Classification and incidence. In benign neoplasms the classification is usually according to tissue of origin and the incidence has no reliable figures for any age, whereas in malignant neoplasms the classification is usually according to cell of origin and the incidence is about 300 cases per 100,000 people, with the disease being predominantly in the middle and older aged. However, certain lesions such as testicular tumors, Hodgkin's disease, and osteogenic sarcoma, do occur in younger age groups.

Predisposing factors. Some carcinogens, such as hydrocarbon compounds, certain heavy metals (arsenic or silicone in asbestos), ionizing radiations, and smoking, are known to predispose to neoplasia. Certain animal experiments show that the early cellular changes attributable to carcinogens are benign and reversible. However, they soon change to become malignant, invasive, and irreversible.

Histology

Capsule. In the benign form the capsule is usually complete and well defined and, as a result, surrounding tissues are only displaced or compressed. But in the malignant form, the capsule is usually incomplete and ill defined or may be absent altogether. As a result, surrounding tissues are invaded in addition to being displaced or compressed.

Tissue. Benign tissue is usually well differentiated and greatly resembles the tissue of origin, but malignant tissue is usually ill defined and may have little resemblance to the tissue of origin. "Anaplastic" tumors are so called because no tissue of origin is deducible from their appearance.

Cells. Benign cells are usually of normal appearance, have slight hyperchromasia, and have an increased number of mitoses, but malignant cells commonly display numerous and abnormal mitotic figures. Their nuclei are hyperchromatic and irregular in size and shape.

Vessels. Vessels in benign tumors are well formed, whereas malignant tumor vessels are usually ill formed. Sometimes malignant tumors display neovascularity, increased capillary network, or increased vascular spaces. Should the tumor outstrip its vascular supply during its growth, the center may be necrotic.

Lymphatics. Lymphatic vessels in benign tumors are well formed and not invaded, but those in malignant ones are frequently poorly formed and often invaded by the growth. As a result, neighboring lymph nodes may be involved.

Rate of growth. Benign tumors are usually slow growing. They may stop after a period or undergo spontaneous regression, but malignant ones are usually rapidly growing. This rate can be measured by the "doubling time," which is defined as the time necessary for the doubling of the number of the cells with each division. Most authors claim that tumors neither grow at a steady rate nor homogeneously. Spontaneous regression rarely occurs, and these incidents when reported are more often in certain types, such as neuroblastoma, malignant melanoma, renal cell carcinoma or breast cancer.

Mode of growth or spread. The majority of benign tumors grow by expansion and compression of surrounding structures. Lymphatic, vascular, or coelomic spread is not known as a rule, even though all malignant tumors generally spread along the same lines. The frequency of spread along one route or the other depends, among other factors, on the histological type and organ of origin. The four common routes of spread are direct, lymphatic, hematological, and coelomic.

DIRECT SPREAD. The malignant tumor invades the surrounding structures and fixes itself to its bed. It may invade lymphatics (causing edema), blood vessels (hemorrhage), nerves (pain and paralysis), or bones (fractures). The invasion is usually related to the rate of growth of the tumor. Organ capsules and arteries are more resistant to this type of spread.

LYMPHATIC SPREAD. The tumor spreads to the draining lymph nodes either by embolism or by lymphatic permeation. Though it is usual for the draining lymph nodes to be involved in some form of systematic spread, sporadic involvement of far nodes is not unknown. The more richly endowed with lymphatics the organ is (such as the posterior third of the tongue), the earlier and wider is the lymphatic spread.

HEMATOLOGICAL SPREAD. As a result of vascular invasion, the tumor spreads widely to distant organs. Those most commonly affected are bones, lungs, liver, and brain. However, no organ is immune.

COELOMIC SPREAD. Malignant cells, when set free in a coelom, such as the peritoneum or pleura, may grow to form seedlings, which may further grow to sheets or sizable tumors associated with accumulation of fluid in the form of ascites or pleural effusion.

Pathological effects. Since the benign tumor grows mainly by expansion, there is compression of surrounding normal structures; for example, pressure on the trachea by a thyroid adenoma causes dyspnea; pressure on the veins by mediastinal teratoma leads to face edema; pressure on the optic nerves by a pituitary adenoma results in blindness because of degeneration of the nerves; and pressure on intracranial draining veins by a meningoma may lead to increased intracranial tension.

However, for malignant tumors, in addition to the pathological effects of compression of surrounding normal structures, invasion leads to a somewhat different picture. Invasion of nerves results in paralysis, such as laryngeal palsy from bronchial carcinoma involving the recurrent laryngeal nerve. Invasion of vessels results in bleeding that may be fatal, such as the invasion of the carotid artery by neck malignancies. Invasion of bone may result in pathological fracture. Lymph node involvement can produce a mass that affects surrounding structures by compression or invasion similar to a primary tumor mass. Distant hematological spread may lead to symptoms dependent on the site of the metastasis. Coelomic spread may result in effusion, whether pleural or peritoneal, and abdominal masses that may lead to intestinal obstruction.

Systemic changes. Systemic changes of benign tumors usually occur in one of the following two conditions: (1) The tumor is formed of secretory cells, such as pancreatic adenoma (insulinoma), which may secrete excessive insulin leading to hypoglycemic symptoms. (2) The tumor is pressing on a hormone-producing organ, leading to its irritation and hormone secretion. More often such pressure results in the inhibition of the hormone secretion, such as pituitary adenoma causing diabetes insipidus as a result of the reduction of antidiuretic hormone.

In addition to the above-described changes, malignant tumors are capable of producing other systemic effects such as those attributable to the *secretion of hormonal substances* by oat cell carcinoma. *Malignant neuropathy* is a syndrome that may result from degenerative changes related to the presence of malignancy per se without specific invasion or pressure on any neurological structure. It occurs in several malignant lesions, particularly bronchial carcinoma and to a lesser extent gastric and ovarian malignancies. The most common changes are peripheral neuropathy, cerebellar degeneration and generalized neuromyopathies. *General deterioration,* loss of appetite, and emaciation may result from malignancy without any specific involvement of the gastrointestinal system or even pain. *Metabolic changes* as a result of malignancy, such as hypercalcemia, is known to occur, especially with advanced bone involvement in metastatic breast carcinoma or multiple myeloma. Hyponatremia occurs with oat cell carcinoma. Changes in the protein metabolism are also known to occur in multiple myeloma, among other diseases.

Changes in tumor. Benign tumors may undergo some changes with the passage of time, such as calcification or hyalinization (uterine myoma). Rarely there may be bleeding in a benign cyst or interference with the blood supply of a tumor because of torsion of a pedicle. Some benign tumors may turn malignant with time.

As malignant tumors grow in a very irregular fashion, the tumor may undergo various changes, because of a lack of proper blood supply such as in necrosis, and break down, a condition that may lead to malignant abscess formation. The abnormal vascular supply may result in bleeding in the lesion, leading to a sudden increase in the tumor size.

Clinical staging. Benign tumors are rarely staged because the tumor is usually localized and its complete removal is curative.

Malignant tumors, on the other hand, are staged according to the degree of spread. Clinical staging helps to give as clear an idea as possible about the natural history of the disease and its prognosis. Consequently, proper staging would help in the choice of the proper line of management. Several systems of staging were evolved. The one that is gaining rapid recognition is the international TNM system.

T stands for tumor. Tumors are classified T1, T2, T3, and T4, according to their size and degree of local invasion. Details are discussed under the proper systems.

N stands for node metastases. They are classified into the following:

- **N1** First station nodes are enlarged, firm, and mobile.
- **N2** Bilateral nodes are enlarged and mobile.
- **N3** Nodes are fixed.

M stands for clinically apparent metastases, which are classified as follows:

- **M0** No metastases are present.
- **M1** Metastases can be present in any organ.

Treatment. Treatment of benign tumors usually means surgery. Radiotherapy is employed only on rare occasions where surgery is not applicable because of the site of the lesion, such as hemangioma in a vertebral body or where surgery is too hazardous, such as in certain cases of pituitary adenoma.

Treatment of malignant tumors usually depends on the stage of the disease. In *localized* tumors, treatment is by surgery or radiotherapy or a combination of both depending on the type of tumor and its site. The duty of the physician is to determine whether treatment is aimed at cure or palliation depending on the extent of the lesion and its natural history. In *widespread disease,* apart from rare lesions, such as some forms of leukemia and lymphomas, the only available treatment for such lesions is palliation, for relieving symptoms or preventing the development of serious complications that may prove fatal if treatment is not instituted.

Prognosis. Benign tumors are usually curable, whereas the prognosis of malignant tumors depends on the clinical stage of the disease; the more advanced the stage, the worse is the prognosis. However, some tumors, such as osteogenic sarcoma, bronchial carcinoma, or esophageal carcinoma, are known by their poor natural history and unfavorable prognosis even in early lesions. Other lesions, such as some cases of thyroid carcinoma or breast carcinoma, have a relatively good prognosis even when advanced. Some of these lesions may be hormone dependent and long survival may result from the correct hormonal balance.

CHAPTER 9

AIR AND FOOD PASSAGES

GENERAL CONSIDERATIONS

In the following paragraphs general characteristics common to air and food passages are discussed. Specifics are detailed under each site later.

Anatomy

Both air and food passages are classified into upper and lower divisions.

Air passages. The *upper air passages* (Fig. 9-1) comprise the nose and paranasal sinuses, pharynx (nasopharynx, oropharynx, and laryngopharynx), larynx, and the upper trachea (extrathoracic). The *lower air passages* are the tracheobronchial tree and alveoli.

Food passages. The *upper food passages* comprise the oral cavity, oropharynx, laryngopharynx (or hypopharynx), and esophagus. The *lower food passages* are the stomach, intestines (including the small intestines and colon), rectum, and anal canal.

Glands. The glands common to both upper air and food passages are the *endocrine glands,* mainly the thyroid and parathyroid. The *exocrine glands* comprise the salivary glands, which are the parotid, submaxillary, and sublingual glands, and mucous glands (spread throughout the whole system). The pancreas is both an endocrine (insulin) and exocrine (digestive enzymes) gland peculiar to the digestive system.

Lymphatic drainage

The lymphatic drainage of the upper air and food passages is almost identical with the following main nodal stations (Fig. 9-2): preauricular lymph nodes, submandibular lymph nodes, submental lymph nodes (midline drain on each side), deep cervical chain (upper, middle, and lower), and the accessory group of nodes (superficial to the accessory nerves). The jugulodigastric nodes are part of the upper deep cervical group.

In the upper passages, lymph usually drains to the nodal station nearest the tumor origin first and then eventually to a corresponding level of the deep cervical chain.

In lower passages, the lymphatics of the tracheobronchial tree drain mainly to the hilar and parahilar nodes. Eventually the mediastinal nodes are involved. The lymphatics of the lower food passages drain first to a station of nodes in the outside covering of the part affected, such as the gastric nodes and pararectal nodes. The

86 Clinical radiation oncology

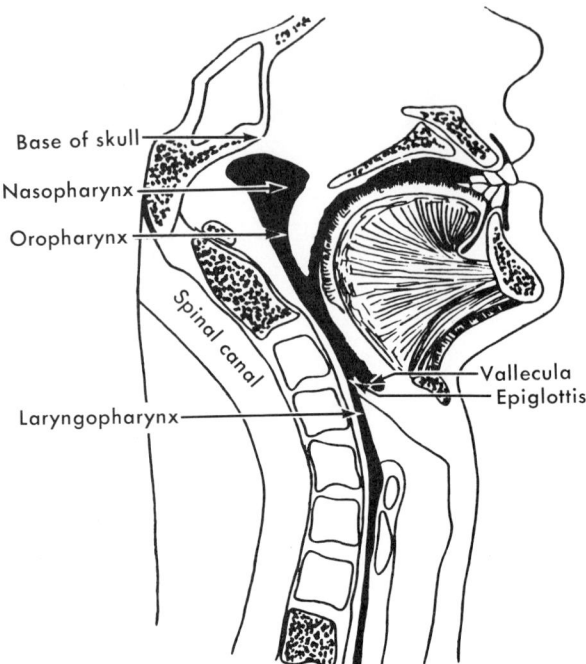

FIG. 9-1. Anatomy of upper air and food passages.

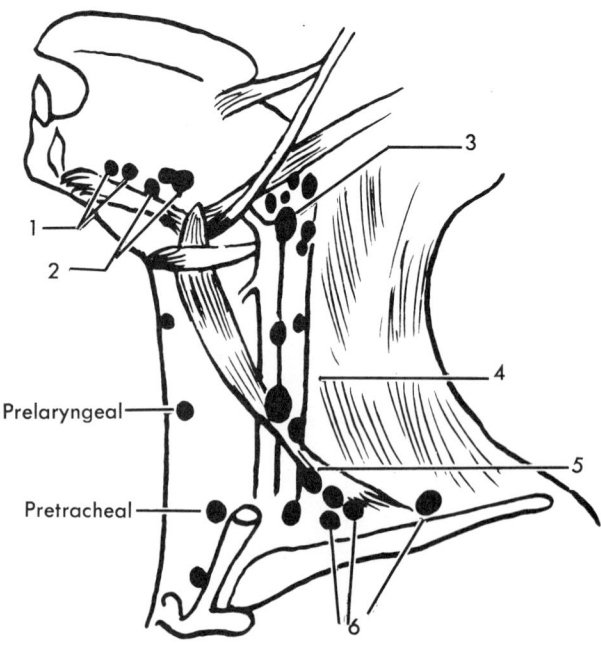

FIG. 9-2. Lymphatics of head and neck. **1**, Submental nodes. **2**, Submandibular nodes. **3**, Jugulodigastric upper deep cervical nodes. **4**, Middle deep cervical nodes. **5**, Lower deep cervical nodes. **6**, Supraclavicular nodes.

second nodal station is situated in the root of the mesentery of the organ. The third station, which is eventually affected, comprises the para-aortic or celiac nodes. Sometimes the major lymph trunks (the thoracic and mediastinal ducts) are involved, with spread to the left supraclavicular nodes.

PATHOLOGICAL CLASSIFICATIONS

Tumors affecting any site depend on the type of the normal mucous membrane lining. Where the tissue is normally stratified (such as the buccal cavity, pharynx, larynx, and esophagus) squamous epithelium, the common lesion, is squamous cell carcinoma; whereas tumors are usually adenocarcinomas when secretory glands are prevalent (intestines and rectum). In regions where lymphoid aggregates are common, such as the tonsils and the posterior third of the tongue, the lymphomatous type of neoplasms may develop.

Tumors affecting the air and food passages are listed as follows, but their relative frequency varies from one site to the other:
1. Squamous cell carcinomas (commoner in upper air and food passages)
2. Adenocarcinomas (commoner in lower food passages)
3. Undifferentiated or anaplastic tumors (oat cell carcinoma is a type common to and characteristic of lung tumors)
4. Lymphoid tissue tumors, such as Hodgkin's disease and non-Hodgkin lymphomas (lymphosarcomas and reticulum cell sarcomas); for more detail see discussion in Chapter 14
5. Mucous and salivary gland tumors
   a. Pleomorphic adenoma or mixed salivary gland tumor (a benign tumor) with a malignant form (malignant mixed tumor or pleomorphic adenocarcinoma)
   b. Adenocarcinomas
   c. Mucoepidermoid tumors
   d. Adenoid cystic carcinomas (cylindromas)
6. Rare tumors (myeloma, rhabdomyosarcoma, angiosarcoma, and malignant melanoma)

PRESENTING SYMPTOMS

Patients usually present with one or more of the following symptoms, but the order of frequency varies according to the site:
1. Symptoms caused by irritation. For example, in the larynx they are cough and hoarseness, whereas in the lower food passages they are diarrhea and nausea.
2. Symptoms caused by obstruction. For example, in the esophagus it is dysphagia, whereas in laryngeal lesions it is stridor. Obstruction of the tracheobronchi produces dyspnea. There may be intestinal obstruction or, in earlier cases, constipation.
3. Symptoms and signs caused by pain. Pain is either localized or referred. Localized pain occurs in oral cavity malignancies with ulceration. Referred pain in the form of earache occurs in advanced lesions of the tongue or floor of the mouth.
4. Symptoms caused by bleeding. In lesions of the esophagus and the stomach, bleeding results in hematemesis, whereas for intestines it is melena. In rectal carcinoma rectal bleeding is a cardinal sign. Carcinoma of the tracheobronchial tree may lead to hemoptysis.
5. Symptoms caused by metastatic spread. For example, in carcinoma of the nasopharynx, a mass of cervical lymph node metastasis may present, or in bronchial carcinoma, a pathological fracture may present.
6. Swelling as in the case of parotid tumors.

INVESTIGATIONS

Investigations include several modalities —roentgenographic, endoscopic, cytological and histopathological.

Roentgenographic methods include plain films (such as chest x-ray films and x-ray films of paranasal sinuses), tomograms, opaque material studies (such as barium swallow, barium enema, bronchograms), and angiograms (such as coeliac selective angiography for gastric and pancreatic lesions).

Endoscopic studies include bronchoscopy, esophagoscopy, mediastinoscopy, laryngoscopy (indirect and direct), and proctosigmoidoscopy.

Cytological studies include sputum examination, bronchial washings, and gastric washings.

Histopathological studies include examination of biopsy material under the light microscope and under the electron microscope on rare occasions.

Exploratory operations (laparotomy, thoracotomy) are carried out when the diagnosis cannot be established by any of the above means.

TREATMENT

Radiotherapy plays a dual role in dealing with tumors of the air and food passages.

Radical

This treatment is aimed at cure. Cure usually takes about 6 weeks and a tumor dose of about 6000 rads. This course of treatment is usually demanding, and patients have to be nursed carefully through it. The volume to be treated, the plan of treatment, and the actual dose depend on the site of the lesion and are discussed separately for each site.

Palliative

Since a large portion of patients suffering from malignant tumors of the air and food passages present in a stage considered to be beyond cure, palliation is the only help medicine may be able to offer. The main symptoms that may be palliated by radiotherapy are the following:

1. *Bleeding.* Radiation is a successful styptic agent, and doses necessary are moderate, about 3000 to 4000 rads in 3 weeks.
2. *Pain.* Pain may have different etiologies upon which the role of and response to radiotherapy depends.
    a. Radiotherapy is most successful in treating bone pain (metastases or direct spread).
    b. Functional pain, such as dysphagia in carcinoma of the piriform fossa or trismus caused by lesions involving the pterygoid fossa may be palliated by radiation. The more advanced the tumor is, the less the quality of palliation, a fact caused by permanent destruction of the muscles carrying the physiological function.
    c. Pain from involvement of nerves by malignant extension does not respond to radiation well although partial relief is almost always achieved.
    d. Pain, caused by capsular distention such as in parotid carcinoma, is relieved by radiotherapy.
3. *Relief of pressure symptoms* caused by a tumor, such as superior vena caval obstruction in advanced carcinoma of the bronchus, respond to radiotherapy very satisfactorily. Other examples include dyspnea caused by thyroid carcinoma and intestinal obstruction caused by enlarged abdominal nodes.
4. *Growth restraint.* When the tumor extent is such that cure is not feasible, radiation can restrain the local growth of the tumor and prevent or delay the development of unpleasant symptoms, such as ulceration and fungation. Examples are recurrent malignant salivary tumors.

In discussing tumors of particular sites, we stress only specific points that depart from those mentioned in general considerations.

TUMORS OF PARANASAL SINUSES

The main paranasal sinuses (Fig. 9-3) affected are the maxillary antrum in about

Air and food passages 89

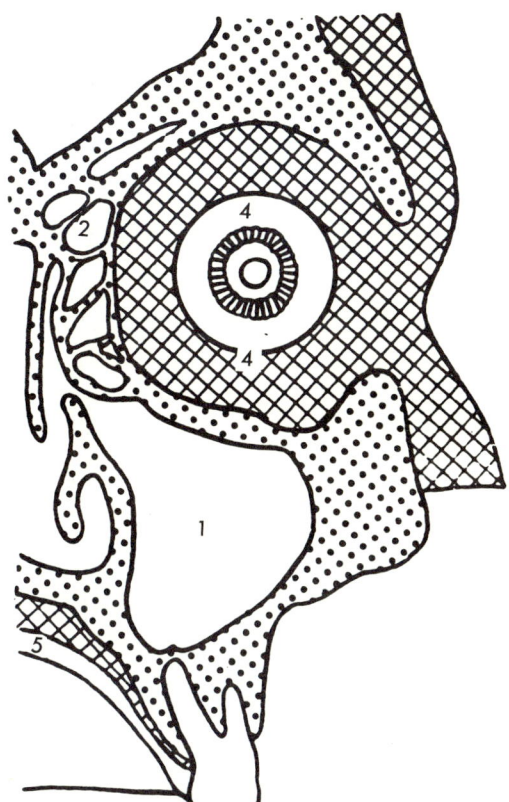

FIG. 9-3. Anatomy of paranasal sinuses: 1, Antrum. 2, Ethmoid cells. 3, Frontal sinus (not shown). 4, Orbit and eye. 5, Palate.

90% of cases and the ethmoid cells in about 8%. Only on rare occasions are the frontal and sphenoidal sinuses the primary sites of origin.

Pathological types

Squamous cell carcinomas, anaplastic carcinomas, and adenocarcinomas are the most common types arranged in order of frequency. Other types are rare.

Incidence

Paranasal sinus tumors form 3% of all head and neck tumors and 0.5% of all malignant tumors.

Spread

The main method of *spread* of these tumors is by *local extension,* which depends on the sinus of origin. Antral tumors may spread in the two following ways according to position: (1) Those of the superior portion may extend medially to the ethmoid cells, superiorly to the orbital floor and the base of skull, anteriorly to the anterior wall of the antrum, and posteriorly to the nasal cavity and nasopharynx; (2) those of the inferior portion may extend anteriorly to the anterior wall of the antrum (and cheek), inferiorly to the palate and alveolus, and posteriorly to the nasopharynx. Evidence of bone destruction is present in half the cases.

Ethmoidal tumors may extend to the contralateral ethmoidal cells and orbital walls, anteriorly to the bridge of the nose, superiorly to the floor of the anterior cranial fossa and the frontal sinus, inferiorly to the maxillary antrum, and posteroinferiorly to the nasopharynx. The sphenoidal sinus may be involved by posterior extension.

Lymphatic spread is relatively late because of the paucity of lymphatics. Nodes affected are mainly the submandibular and upper deep cervical chain.

Distant spreads are fairly late.

Clinical staging

Clinical staging of tumors of the paranasal sinuses is rather difficult. A knowledge of the histology and extent of spread of disease is often adequate in directing proper therapy. An attempt at staging was described by Ohngren when he divided the maxillary antrum by a line extending from the inner canthus to the angle of the lip into two portions—the anteroinferior and the posterosuperior. Lesions in the latter portion have a poor prognosis.

Treatment policy

Best results are achieved by a combination of surgery and radiotherapy. The regime for antral tumors is usually as follows:

1. Caldwell Luc operation whereby a drill hole is established in the incisor fossa. It has the following functions:

it serves as a biopsy site; drains the sinus from sloughs, infections, and secretions; and serves as a window to inspect the response to treatment.

2. A course of radiotherapy (external irradiation).
3. Radical antrectomy with detailed postoperative biopsy of various limits of surgical excision (walls of the established cavity).
4. Complementary radiotherapy to any residual disease.

Treatment of ethmoidal tumors is along the same lines, but surgery is more limited because a radical operation would mean the loss of both eyes and generally it is rarely feasible. The main method of treatment is therefore radiotherapy with only limited surgical procedures.

Technique of radiotherapy

For external irradiation, cobalt beam or supervoltage beam is the method of choice. An example plan of treatment is shown in Fig. 9-4, where a two-wedge arrangement is employed. The dose arrived at is usually within 6000 to 6500 rads in 6 to 6½ weeks. The volume treated should include the antrum, ethmoids, nose, orbit to base of skull, and palate. The eye is fully or partially protected, if possible, depending on the extent of disease.

Supplementary radiotherapy is given by the method most appropriate to treat the residual disease. This is done either by a mold with radioactive sources installed where there is residual disease or by a radioactive implant (gold grains or radon seeds). External irradiation is rarely indicated, but an electron beam may be successfully employed to a small volume.

Prognosis

About one third of the patients live free from disease for 5 years. The usual problems are directly caused by local recurrence

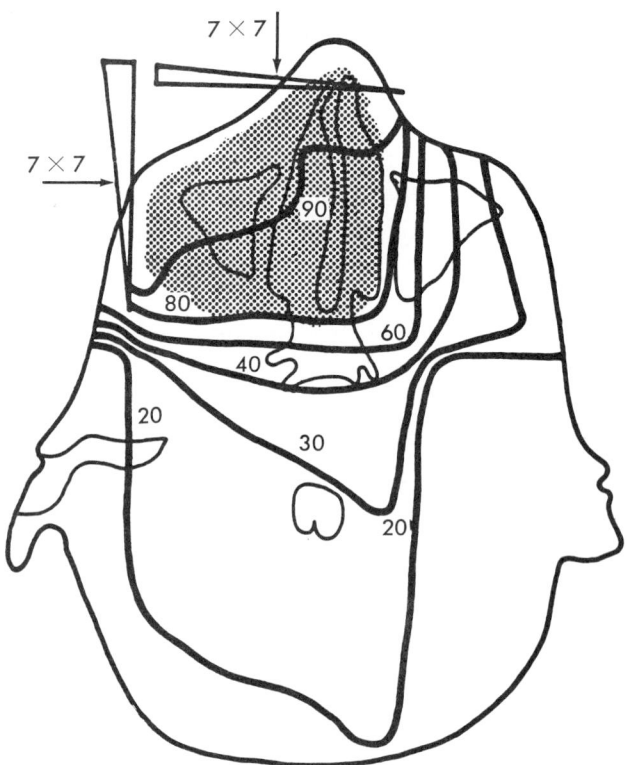

FIG. 9-4. Wedge plan for treatment of maxillary antrum.

and its complications, which are infection, bleeding, and involvement of adjacent vital structures (contents of the anterior cranial fossa).

NASOPHARYNGEAL TUMORS
Incidence

Nasopharyngeal tumors are especially common in Chinese. The peak age incidence is the fifth decade of life. It is twice as common in males.

Pathological types

The most common pathological types are squamous cell carcinoma, anaplastic carcinoma, lymphosarcoma, adenocarcinoma, in order of frequency.

Spread (Fig. 9-1)

The tumor extends *locally* to the base of the skull and affects the cranial nerves and their foramina. The third to sixth nerves are the most vulnerable, giving rise to the "retropharyngeal syndrome." Lateral extension in the parapharyngeal space toward the jugular foramen affects the ninth to twelfth cranial nerves, causing the "retrosphenoidal syndrome of Villaret." Anterior extension may involve the choana, nasal cavity, ethmoidal cells, maxillary antrum, and orbit.

Lymphatic spread is common and early, affecting usually the whole cervical chain (75% to 85% of cases), and is not uncommonly bilateral (35% of cases). The jugulodigastric nodal station is the one frequently involved. Spinal accessory and posterior triangle nodes are frequently involved—a unique feature of nasopharyngeal cancer.

Distant spread is relatively late affecting mainly lungs and bones.

Clinical picture

Symptoms of cranial nerve involvement are a common presenting picture and include diplopia caused by paralysis of oculomotor nerves, pain caused by involvement of the fifth nerve, or trophic corneal ulceration caused by loss of the sensory component of the fifth cranial nerve.

Nasal obstruction and epistaxis complete the usual presenting picture. Enlarged cervical nodes is a frequent reason for a patient to seek medical advice.

Treatment policy

Radiotherapy is the treatment of choice, and surgery is limited to the palliative procedures, such as tarsorrhaphy to compensate for oculomotor paralysis, and the occasional excision of metastatic lymph nodes, if the primary tumor is controlled successfully. Exploration by palatal fenestration may become necessary.

Technique of radiotherapy

External irradiation is the prime modality, with interstitial implantation reserved for residual or recurrent disease. As with all head and neck cases the main problem is to give a high dose to the tumor volume without overirradiating the spinal cord and other adjacent vital structures such as the

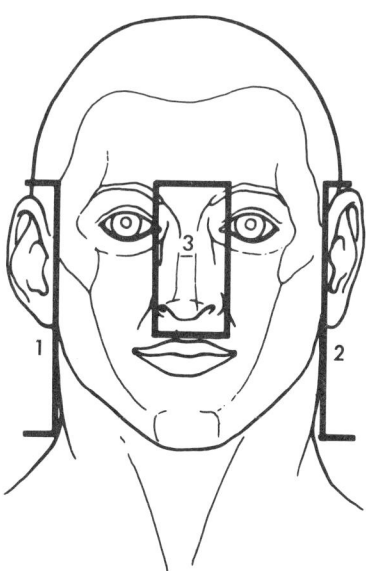

Fig. 9-5. Fields used in the treatment of carcinoma of the nasopharynx. **1** and **2**, Two lateral fields and an anterior one, **3**. This third one is particularly used when the tumor extends into the nasal cavity.

eye. Cobalt or supervoltage beams are utilized for their beneficial characteristics (deeper penetration, less skin reaction, more homogeneous dose, and less bone absorption). The fields used are shown in Fig. 9-5.

Prognosis

The prognosis is usually bad. Only about 25% to 35% of the patients live for 5 years free of disease. Women have a better prognosis.

CARCINOMA OF LARYNX

Carcinoma of the larynx represents less than 2% of all cancers. The results of treatment are very good, with a 5-year cure of early cases as high as 90% in glottic lesions. It is more frequent in men and has a strong relation to heavy smoking and drinking. Leukoplakia is accepted by some as a precursor. The peak age incidence is the fifth and sixth decades of life.

Anatomy

The larynx is divided into the following three regions (Fig. 9-6): (1) glottic, comprising the true vocal cords and anterior commissure; (2) supraglottic, comprising the false cords, ventricles, aryepiglottic folds, arytenoids, and the epiglottis; and (3) subglottic, or the region below the true cords.

Clinical picture

The clinical picture varies from the frequent symptom of hoarseness of the voice to dysphagia in the supraglottic lesions and to pain, which may be local or referred to the ear. Pain is somewhat ominous, as it denotes advanced disease. Dyspnea and stridor are also symptoms of advanced disease. Cervical lymphadenopathy may be the presenting picture for subglottic lesions.

Spread

Local spread leads to infiltration of deeper structures, resulting in fixation of the cord or hemilarynx. A glottic ulcer may extend from one cord to the other, causing a "kiss" ulcer or involvement of the anterior commissure. Eventually the tumor spreads from one anatomical region to the other

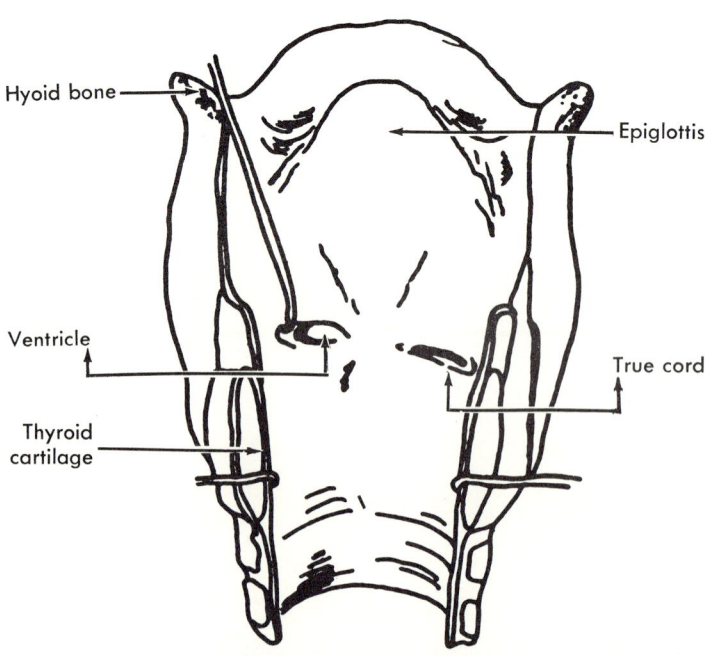

Fig. 9-6. Anatomy of larynx.

TABLE 9-1. Definitions of TNM categories for larynx classified according to anatomic site of origin as divided into three regions*

Supraglottic	Glottic	Subglottic
Posterior surface of epiglottis (including tip), aryepiglottic fold, arytenoid, ventricular bands (false cords), ventricular cavities (right and left)	True vocal cords (right and left), anterior glottic commissure	Subglottic region, exclusive of undersurface of true cords

TIS Carcinoma in situ

T1 Tumor limited to one anatomic region within larynx with normal mobility

T1a Tumor limited to one site

Supraglottic	Glottic	Subglottic
Tumor confined to laryngeal surface of epiglottis, or to an aryepiglottic fold or arytenoid, or to a ventricular cavity or a ventricular band	Tumor confined to one vocal cord and mobility of cord remains normal	Tumor limited to one side of subglottic region, exclusive of undersurface of cord

T1b Tumor involving more than one site

Supraglottic	Glottic	Subglottic
Tumor arising on epiglottis, aryepiglottic fold, arytenoid, ventricular cavity or band, and extending to involve one or more of adjacent supraglottic sites	Tumor involving both cords with normal mobility of cords	Tumor extending to two sides of subglottic region, exclusive of undersurface of cords

T2 Tumor extending beyond one anatomic region but confined to larynx without fixation

Supraglottic	Glottic	Subglottic
Tumor of epiglottis and/or aryepiglottic folds, arytenoids, ventricular cavity or bands, and extending onto cords	Tumor extending from cords either to subglottic region or to supraglottic region, i.e., to ventricular bands or ventricles (includes those patients with normal and/or impaired mobility of cords)	Tumor involving subglottic region and extending onto cords

T3 Tumor as in T1 or T2 with fixation of larynx

Supraglottic	Glottic	Subglottic
Tumor limited to larynx with fixation and/or destruction or other evidence of deep invasion	Tumor limited to larynx with fixation of cords	Tumor limited to larynx with fixation of cords

T4 Tumor extending beyond larynx

Supraglottic	Glottic	Subglottic
Tumors of supraglottis that extend beyond larynx, i.e., extension to piriform sinus, postcricoid region, vallecula, or base of tongue, etc.	Tumors of cords that extend beyond larynx, i.e., into cartilage, to piriform sinus, or to postcricoid region, etc.	Tumors of subglottis that extend beyond larynx, i.e., extension to trachea, skin, or postcricoid region, etc.

*American Joint Committee for Cancer Staging and End Results Reporting, 1972 revision.

Continued.

TABLE 9-1. Definitions of TNM categories for larynx classified according to anatomic site of origin as divided into three regions—cont'd

Metastasis to cervical nodes

- N0   Cervical nodes not palpable
- N1   Palpable cervical lymph nodes, homolateral, not fixed
- N1a   Metastasis not suspected
- N1b   Metastasis suspected
- N2   Palpable bilateral, contralateral, or midline lymph nodes, not fixed
- N2a   Metastasis not suspected
- N2b   Metastasis suspected
- N3   Fixed cervical lymph nodes, metastasis suspected

Distant metastasis

- M0   No distant metastasis
- M1   Clinical or radiographic

Staging—invasive cancers of larynx

			Cumulative survival at five years	
			Glottic	Supraglottic
Stage I	T1	N0, N1a or N2a M0	94%	91%
Stage II	T2	N0, N1a or N2a M0	85%	82%
Stage III	T3	N0, N1a or N2a M0 65%⎫		74%⎫
	T4	N0, N1a or N2a M0 40%⎬ 59%		55%⎬ 49%
	T1 T2 T3 or T4	⎫		45%⎭
	N1b or N2b	⎬ M0 54%⎭		
Stage IV	T1 T2 T3 or T4 N3 M0	⎫		
	or	⎬	9%	9%
	T1 T2 T3 or T4			
	N0 N1 N2 N3 M1	⎭		

and to surrounding structures such as cartilage, muscle, or nerves.

Lymphatic spread of glottic cancer is unusual, but it is more frequent in supraglottic and subglottic tumors. The upper and middle deep cervical nodes are those most commonly involved.

Distant metastases in laryngeal carcinoma occurs infrequently.

Clinical staging

The American Joint Committee on Cancer Staging and End Result Reporting devised the revised (1972) classification of the larynx shown in Table 9-1. Within each of the three categories the extent of the disease is defined according to the TNM (*T*, primary tumor; *N*, regional lymph nodes; *M*, distant metastasis) categories.

Treatment policy

Although results of treatment of early cases by either surgery or radiotherapy are equally good, those of late cases are more favorable with radiotherapy than with surgery. However, recent work indicates that a combination of both may be the treatment of choice. Surgery usually means laryngectomy and loss of voice and is indicated in the following conditions: (1) radioresistant cases, where the lesions did not respond favorably to radiotherapy; (2) local recurrence, and (3) cervical lymph node metastases after preoperative radiation.

Technique of radiotherapy

The beams used are either ^{60}Co rays or supervoltage x rays with small field wedge

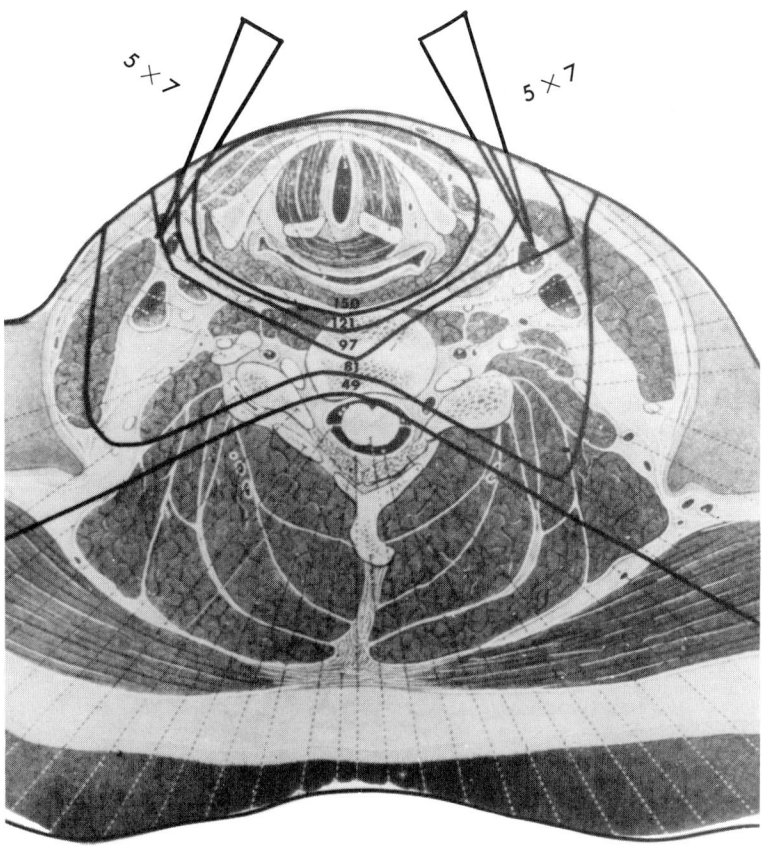

FIG. 9-7. Plan to treat larynx.

arrangements (Fig. 9-7). However, in lesions of supraglottic or subglottic lesions larger fields are used to include the immediate draining lymph nodes. The dose aimed at is about 6000 to 7000 rads in 6 to 7 weeks, with the higher dose reserved for advanced lesions. In case of postoperative radiotherapy the dose has to be modified.

Complications of radiotherapy are particularly noticeable in advanced lesions with cartilage involvement. The main complication is edema, which may lead to obstruction of the airway, necessitating tracheostomy. However, careful treatment planning, elimination of infection, and sources of chronic irritation (smoking, talking) would limit such incidents only to the very advanced cases.

Late neurological complications may occur when fields irradiating large segments of the spinal cord to high doses are used.

Prognosis

At least three fourths of the patients suffering from early carcinoma of the larynx live free of disease for 5 years, but only about 40% of the late cases do so. On the whole, about two thirds of all patients treated survive 5 years free of disease. Glottic tumors classified as T1 or T2 are indeed curable in 80% to 90% of the cases. Those patients treated with radiotherapy continue to enjoy a normal voice.

CARCINOMA OF BRONCHUS

The incidence of this tumor doubled between 1950 and 1965, and the number of resulting deaths is increasing at an alarming rate in recent years. It is strongly related to cigarette smoking and exposure to coal tars and asbestos. Miners involved with radioactive ores and refiners of nickel are considered to be high-risk groups. The disease is more prevalent in males (10:1), with the prevalent age incidence being during the fifth and sixth decades of life.

The tumor usually originates in the main bronchi and less commonly in the smaller ones. Alveoli are rarely the site of origin. Consequently most of the tumors could be detected by bronchoscopy, except if they affect inaccessible bronchi.

Pathological types

The most common are squamous cell, oat cell, and anaplastic carcinomas. Adenocarcinomas are uncommon and are usually located peripherally. Mucous gland tumors are rare and originate from mucous glands in large bronchi.

Clinical types

There are two major types—the central and the peripheral. The central type arises from the main tracheobronchial tree, usually seen on x rays near the lung hilum. An accessory peripheral shadow caused by collapsed lung tissue may exist. The peripheral type arises from terminal bronchi or alveoli. These are rare tumors and may spread to the pleura relatively early. This type is more common in nonsmokers and females and is usually an adenocarcinoma. Pancoast's tumor (pulmonary sulcus tumor), affecting the lung apex, is a type of peripheral tumor, but it is commonly a squamous cell carcinoma.

Spread

Locally these tumors extend by infiltrating bronchial walls or growing intraluminally. Eventually they infiltrate the surrounding lung tissue, or adjacent diaphragmatic or parietal pleura, resulting in pain or effusion. Occasionally the pericardium is involved with or without effusion.

Lymphatic spread is usually early and wide, affecting the bronchial, tracheobronchial, and carinal nodes. Eventually mediastinal nodes are involved, and their involvement may lead to superior mediastinal obstruction.

Distant metastases occur early. The organs commonly affected are bones, brain, liver, and adrenals.

Clinical picture

Patients usually present late with fairly advanced disease. Cough, hemoptysis, anorexia, loss of weight, and symptoms of superior mediastinal obstruction form the commonest presenting clinical picture. Rare, but nevertheless important, symptoms are attributable to extrapulmonary manifestations.

These manifestations include metabolic and hormonal abnormalities resulting in hypercalcemia (weakness, lassitude), Cushing's syndrome (see glossary), increased secretions of estrogens (gynecomastia), excessive antidiuretic hormone (edema and water retention), and carcinoid syndrome (diarrhea, palpitation, and flushing).

Peripheral as well as cerebellar neuropathies may be the presenting picture. The former causes pins-and-needles paresthesia in a glove-and-stocking distribution. The latter results in incoordination, weakness, and loss of muscle tone. Clubbing and hypertrophic osteoarthropathy (bone and periosteal reaction) represent a skeletal manifestation. Vascular abnormalities, represented by migratory thrombophlebitis and endocarditis, may also prevail.

Investigations

In addition to investigations discussed in general considerations, scalene node biopsy is positive in about 20% of the cases and is particularly valuable when biopsy through bronchoscopy is not possible or negative. In the cases where superior mediastinal obstruction is the presenting clinical picture, superior venacavography usually confirms the diagnosis (Fig. 9-8) and often demon-

Air and food passages 97

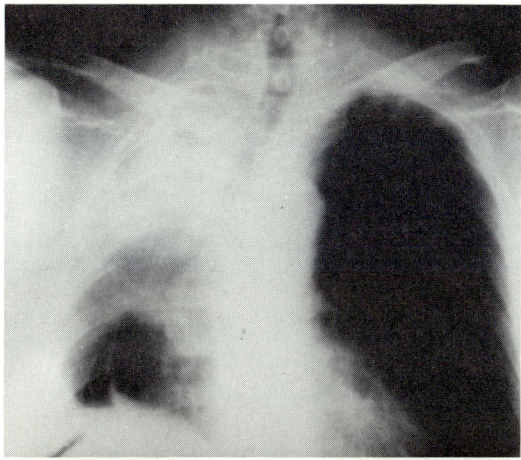
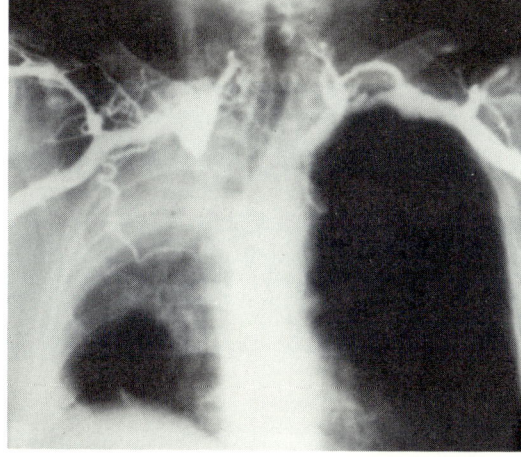

FIG. 9-8. Roentgenogram of superior vena cava showing caval obstruction and filling of collaterals.

strates the level of obstruction. Lung scan is claimed to help delineate the extent of the disease, and it can indicate resectability, or otherwise.

Treatment policy

Treatment is generally governed by the extent of the lesion, its histology, and the general condition of the patient. In case of squamous cell carcinoma and adenocarcinoma, surgical excision, preferably by lobectomy, is the method of choice whenever feasible (when there is a localized lesion and the patient is a good operative risk). However, if resection is not possible because of site of the lesion (such as being too near the carina or in the main trachea) or because the patient is a poor operative risk (such as with poor respiratory functions), a radical course of radiotherapy is the next alternative. In cases of oat cell carcinoma or anaplastic carcinoma, radiotherapy is the method of choice even in surgically resectable lesions because the tumor is highly radiosensitive and the volume of tissues treated usually includes the draining lymph nodes.

Generally, since a good number of cases (45%) are advanced on presentation, cure is not possible and radiotherapy is the method of choice for palliation.

Technique of radiotherapy

External irradiation, usually with the cobalt beam or supervoltage machine is the method of choice because deeper penetration is needed. Larger fields are usually utilized. The dose aimed at depends on the goal of treatment and the histology of the lesions.

Oat cell carcinomas are adequately controlled by a dose of 4500 rads in 4½ weeks, whereas higher doses are required for squamous cell carcinoma or adenocarcinoma. Split course techniques (see glossary) are claimed to have higher survivals in the first two posttreatment years. A dose of about 4000 rads in about 4 weeks is considered adequate for palliation of hemoptysis, superior vena canal obstruction, pain, and dysphagia in over three fourths of cases treated.

Complications of radiotherapy

Pulmonary fibrosis and its sequelae, as a result of radiation pneumonitis, are rather frequent and may lead to respiratory insufficiency. Radiation myelitis may occur, especially in those fortunate enough to live more than 1 year.

Prognosis

The general outlook for this disease is very grim. The overall 5-year survival rate is less than 5% in the best hands. The usual cause of death is distant spread (brain or visceral metastases), in addition to general debility caused by the disease. The best results are in those patients who present with small resectable lesions (usually squamous cell carcinomas). The 5-year survival in this group of patients is about 20% to 30%.

Palliation is highly successful in cases of hemoptysis, bone pain, and superior vena caval obstruction. On the other hand pain from Pancoast's tumors or symptoms resulting from nerve paralysis (such as hoarseness of voice) are seldom relieved.

CARCINOMA OF TONGUE AND ORAL CAVITY

Carcinoma of the oral cavity is most prevalent in the *male* (4:1). The disease is most common in the sixth decade of life. In about 10% of patients suffering from oral carcinoma there is evidence of multicentric origin as an expression of a basically abnormal mucosa. Tobacco smoking, chronic alcoholism, chronic irritation, and Plummer-Vinson syndrome (see glossary) may be *predisposing factors* to oral carcinoma. The oral cavity includes the floor of the mouth, tongue, buccal mucosa (cheek), gingiva, and palate. However, most of our discussion is concentrated on carcinoma of the tongue because it is the most common cancer of the oral cavity, highly lethal, and of special interest to the radiotherapist.

Pathological types

The main types in order of frequency are squamous cell carcinoma (90%), mucous gland tumors, and lymphomatous tumors, which are commoner in the posterior third or base of the tongue.

Spread

Locally the lesions spread to other parts of the tongue, floor of mouth, faucial pillars, and tonsils.

Lymphatic spread occurs relatively early, with a rapid rate of growth. The following nodal stations are involved in order of frequency: ipsilateral jugulodigastric, upper deep cervical, and submandibular nodes. The contralateral nodes and the rest of the cervical chain follow. Tumors of the posterior third of the tongue spread to lymph nodes early and often present with bilateral nodal metastases.

Distant metastases occur relatively late.

Clinical picture

Early lesions have minimal symptoms. However, pain in various forms, such as denture discomfort, local soreness, painful mastication, or dysphagia, is often the presenting picture. Advanced lesions may cause earache. Cervical lymph node enlargement is reported in about half the cases.

Clinical classification depends on the extent of the disease. The classification suggested by the International Union Against Cancer is summarized as follows:

T Primary tumor
T1 Tumor measuring 2 cm. or less in its largest dimension; strictly superficial or exophytic
T2 Tumor measuring 2 cm. or less in its largest dimension with minimal infiltration in depth
T3 Tumor measuring more than 2 cm. in its largest dimension, or tumor with deep infiltration irrespective of its size
T4 Tumor involving other anatomical structures, such as muscle or bone, extending to more than one neighboring region
N Regional lymph nodes
N0 No palpable lymph nodes
N1 Movable homolateral lymph nodes
N2 Movable contralateral or bilateral lymph nodes
N3 Fixed homolateral or bilateral lymph nodes
M Distant metastasis
M0 No evidence of distant metastasis
M1 Distant metastasis

Treatment policy

Treatment depends on the extent of the disease or clinical staging. Early cases can be treated successfully either with surgery or radiotherapy (usually radium implant). Surgery is simpler in lesions of the tip of tongue and particularly indicated where there is evidence of widespread mucous membrane changes (leukoplakia, or chronic glossitis) or for radiotherapy failures. Management of regional nodes is somewhat controversial; they are either watched closely or an immediate block dissection (dissection of the regional neck nodes) is carried out. Advocates of the latter method claim that nodal metastases occur in close to 25% of these patients. Furthermore, block dissection is preferred when the patients live in a rural area where regular follow-up is not feasible. Radiotherapy is claimed to control lymph node metastases equally well, through the utilization of external irradiation (supervoltage) up to a dose of 5000 to 6000 rads per 5 to 6 weeks. In *advanced cases* the results of either radiotherapy or surgery alone are rather disappointing. Over 50% of patients presenting with lesions over 2 cm. in diameter suffer from nodal metastases. Perhaps the best results are obtained by a combination of both. Generally surgery is chosen to control lymph nodes after preoperative radiotherapy, whereas radiotherapy is often effective in dealing with the tongue lesion. Close cooperation between the surgeon and the radiotherapist accompanied by individual planning for each case is necessary to achieve the best results.

The technique of radiation to the tongue utilizes external irradiation with wedge fields or weighted parallel opposing fields, which may be followed by a limited radium implant when indicated.

Carcinomas of the oropharynx

The oropharynx is composed of the soft palate and faucial arches anterolaterally, the posterior third of the tongue anteroinferiorly, the tonsils and lateral pharyngeal wall laterally, and the posterior pharyngeal wall posteriorly (Fig. 9-1). The sites most commonly affected are the posterior third of the tongue and the tonsils.

Tumors of the posterior third or base of the tongue are fairly advanced on presentation with lymph node metastasis in over half the cases. Radical surgery will necessitate laryngectomy and partial pharyngectomy in most cases. This extensive and mutilating surgery is not rewarded by improved results. Moreover, tumors in this region are reported to be more radiosensitive. Consequently radiation is the method of choice. External irradiation by opposing fields to a dose of 6000 to 6500 rads for 6 to 7 weeks is the routine technique. The volume treated includes bilateral nodes, often encompassing all the cervical chain.

Prognosis

Although the results of early cases are generally satisfactory (with a 5-year survival rate of about 65%), the results of treatment of patients presenting with lymph node involvement are often disappointing (about 16% with a 5-year survival rate).

Tonsillar tumors

Tonsillar tumors account for 10% of all head and neck tumors. There is a relatively high incidence of lymphoepithelial tumors, but a majority are still squamous cell carcinoma. Tonsillar carcinomas spread to lymph nodes early, with 70% of patients presenting with metastatic nodes. The first draining node is the jugulodigastric and upper deep cervical chain. Tumors extend locally to involve the faucial pillars, the base of the tongue, and the lateral pharyngeal wall. They may involve the soft palate. With such extensive disease the incidence of contralateral nodes is high (30% to 35%). Both the tonsil and its first draining node are adjacent and form one volume, a fact that facilitates radiotherapy techniques. Tonsillar tumors are radiosensitive, and results of treatment by radiotherapy alone are usually good. External irradiation is the method of choice, and the dose aimed at is 6500 to 7000 rads in 6½ to 7 weeks delivered through weighted opposing fields. Nodes are given the same dose if they are grossly involved; however, the dose is reduced to 5000 rads in 5 weeks if they are not palpable (subclinical disease). Radiotherapy complications include mucous membrane atrophy, dryness of the mouth, and on rare occasions bone necrosis. Complications seem to be related to the extent of disease, the fields employed, and the dose given. Surgery is applicable with good results if the tumor is limited with no extension to any of the surrounding structures. This type of early case is rare. The 5-year survival figure of early cases is about 58%, whereas it is 25% to 39% if the lymph nodes are involved.

TUMORS OF HYPOPHARYNX
Anatomical sites

The hypopharynx is composed of the piriform fossa, the posterior pharyngeal wall, and the postcricoid region.

Tumors of the piriform fossa. Although tumors of the piriform fossa are actually part of the hypopharynx, their problems are similar to the supraglottic lesions. For example, squamous cell carcinoma is the commonest *pathological* type and the tumor *spreads* early to surrounding regions, such as the posterior pharyngeal wall, arytenoid, and aryepiglottic fold. Cervical esophagus involvement may result from extension to parapharyngeal lymphatics. The *clinical picture* includes difficulty in swallowing, with consequent loss of weight and deterioration in the patient's general condition. Hoarseness occurs late. As the lesion spreads to cervical lymph nodes early (middle deep cervical station), a mass in the neck may be the presenting picture. *Treatment* by surgery usually entails partial pharyngectomy and often pharyngolaryngectomy and permanent tracheostomy with consequent loss of voice. Treatment by radiotherapy may yield good results, especially if the tumor is exophytic, is situated superiorly, and has not invaded cartilage or extended to the postcricoid region. Radiotherapy is applied by external irradiation and the dose aimed at is 6500 rads in 6½ weeks. If preoperative or postoperative radiation is contemplated, the fields and dose should be duly modified. *Prognosis*, on the whole, is not very good, as the cases are fairly advanced when presenting. Moreover, even with successful local control, patients continue to die with distant metastases.

Postcricoid carcinoma. Postcricoid carcinoma is the only tumor in the head and neck that is more *common in females*. Chronic anemia and atrophied lingual mucous membrane (Plummer-Vinson syndrome) are known to be *predisposing factors*. Patients usually *present with dysphagia*, which leads to rapid deterioration in the patient's general condition. Tumors are usually locally advanced when presenting for treatment. *Results* of surgery or radiotherapy are very disappointing, only 1 in 10 of the treated patients live for 5 years. Radiotherapy is usually applied by external irradiation with a cobalt beam, utilizing a treatment plan similar to that employed in cases of tumors of the cervical esophagus.

CARCINOMA OF ESOPHAGUS

This disease is characterized by a rather gloomy picture whether during the patient's life or the ultimate prognosis.

Incidence

The *incidence* of esophageal carcinoma is highest in Japan, whereas in Puerto Rico its occurrence is four times that of the continental United States. It is predominant in males (3:1) and 90% of cases occur after 50 years of age. Plummer-Vinson syndrome, achalasia, or hiatus hernia may play a *predisposing role*. A history of alcoholism and liver cirrhosis is encountered frequently.

Anatomical consideration

The esophagus is essentially a muscle tube 25 cm. long and is divided arbitrarily into three parts (Fig. 9-9):

1. Upper third or cervical esophagus extends from esophageal introitus (lower level of cricoid cartilage) to the upper border of aortic arch. It is affected in 20% of the cases.
2. Middle third extends down to just below the tracheal bifurcation and is affected in about a third of the cases.

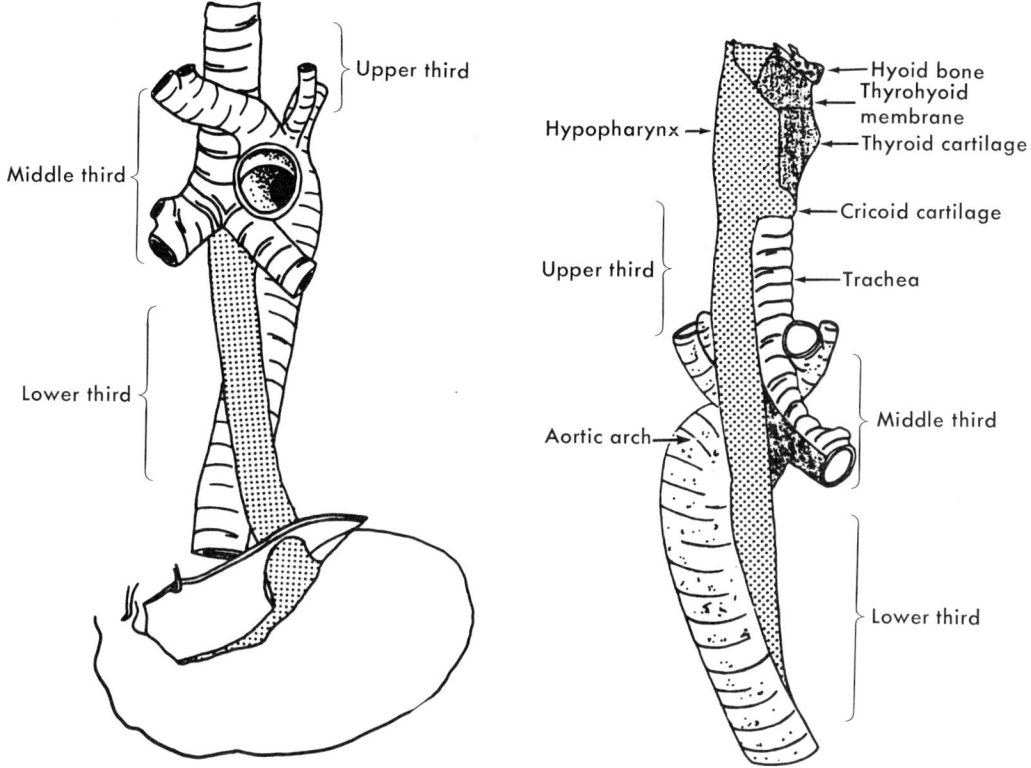

FIG. 9-9. Anatomy of esophagus.

3. Lower third extends down to the cardia and is affected in the remaining 40%.

Pathological types

The *pathological types* include squamous cell carcinoma, usually poorly differentiated, and adenocarcinoma, which arises more commonly in the lower third and is claimed to originate in ectopic gastric mucosa. Other rare tumors include malignant lymphomas, rhabdomyosarcomas, and carcinosarcomas.

Spread

The esophagus has no serosal covering and therefore tumors can extend *locally* along the longitudinal axis (in the ulcerative type) or circumferentially (in the annular type) or toward the lumen (in the cauliflower type). Submucosal infiltration can occur 4 to 7 cm. beyond the apparent clinical border. Invasion of surrounding structures such as mediastinal contents (trachea, great vessels, and nerves) happens early because of the relative thinness of the esophageal wall. The pericardium or mediastinal pleura may also be involved.

Lymphatic spread occurs early and to a wide extent. It is claimed that close to 90% of the lesions over 5 cm. in length have wide nodal metastases. The first draining nodes are the paraesophageal and the mediastinal nodes. The ultimate spread depends on the site of the lesion, being the celiac nodes (below diaphragm) in the lower esophagus or the cervical nodes in the upper esophagus.

Distant metastases are directed mainly to the liver and to the lungs and bones to a lesser extent.

Clinical picture

The presenting symptom is invariably dysphagia followed by vomiting, dehydration and marked loss of weight. Consequently the patient's general condition deteriorates, a fact that would preclude radical therapy with its strains. Pain, laryngeal nerve palsy and anemia are late findings.

Treatment policy

Treatment will vary according to the anatomical site of the tumor.

Upper third lesions are treated by radiotherapy, since radical surgery would entail total esophagectomy, a major procedure that is rarely feasible and carries with it a high mortality.

Middle third carcinomas are managed by various combinations of surgery and radiotherapy. Preoperative radiotherapy followed by surgical excision was employed with good results by the Japanese surgeon Nakayama* in a highly selected group of cases. Pearson† using radiotherapy alone (5000 rads in 4 weeks) showed better results than that attained by esophagectomy.

Cancers of the *lower third* are invariably treated with partial esophagectomy, gastrectomy with a jejunal loop to bridge the gap. The stomach is removed because the tumor may extend into the esophageal wall down to the stomach.

These broad lines are often modified according to the general condition of the patient and extent of the disease. Generally a good percentage of patients are incurable on presentation. Palliation is the only feasible goal in the majority of patients and is readily achieved by radiotherapy.

---

*Nakayama, K., Yazawa, C., Kobayashi, S., et al.: [Preoperative irradiation of cancer—its theory and practice, with special reference to esophageal cancer], Surg. Ther. (Osaka) 18:327, 1968.

†Pearson, J. G.: The value of radiotherapy in the management of esophageal cancer, Am. J. Roentgen, 105:500, March 1969.

Technique of radiotherapy

Radiotherapy is usually applied by a cobalt beam or supervoltage beam. The plan of treatment varies according to region involved. The length of the field is usually about 15 cm. The dose aimed at is 5000 to 6000 rads in 5 to 6 weeks.

When applying radiotherapy to this region, one must avoid overirradiating normal surrounding structures, such as the spinal cord, the trachea, and the lung.

Complications of radiotherapy

Early complications such as increasing dysphagia during and immediately after treatment are caused by mucous membrane reaction. Consequently, the patient needs a great amount of nursing care and perhaps a tube feeding or hyperalimentation during treatment.

Late complications include esophageal stenosis from the fibrosis occuring after irradiation. The patient may need esophageal dilatation. Myelopathy and paraplegia are late sequelae.

Prognosis

Generally the prognosis is bad, and this is very much related to patients presenting with advanced disease. Less than 10% of patients live for 5 years, but results of treatment of the cervical esophagus are somewhat better, about 20% to 25%.

PLACE OF RADIOTHERAPY IN TREATMENT OF STOMACH AND COLONIC TUMORS

Radiotherapy is the method of choice in treating *lymphosarcoma of the stomach,* especially if the tumor, which is usually radiosensitive, has spread widely by the time of laparotomy so that radical surgery is precluded. However if the tumor is localized with no nodal metastases, surgery may be curative, especially if the lesion occurs in the intestines or colon.

External irradiation is the method used in view of the big volume that should be treated and the dose aimed at is 4000 to

4500 rads in about 5 weeks. Results of treatment are usually gratifying.

Palliative radiotherapy is indicated in cases of advanced painful or bleeding *stomach carcinomas,* which are treated by external irradiation to a modest dose, such as 4000 rads in 5 weeks.

The role of radiotherapy in the treatment of *carcinoma of the rectum* is attracting more attention recently. Present studies show a beneficial effect of preoperative radiotherapy by reduction of the incidence of nodal metastases and increasing the percentage of subsequent successful resection of the primary. Postoperative radiotherapy may have a role in the treatment of certain stages of rectal carcinoma. Radiation is also successful in controlling recurrences, especially where limited in size. The palliative effect of radiotherapy in advanced cases is well recognized in controlling bleeding, pain, a fistula, or ulceration. Peritoneal and serosal seedings from carcinomas of the stomach or intestines lead to *malignant ascites* and can be treated by intraperitoneal radioactive colloidal gold or phosphorus (^{32}P), but this method is only useful if the seedings are minute, preferably microscopical. *Metastatic spread* to the spine or nerve roots is usually treated with radiotherapy to control pain. Palliation is limited in case of root pain.

Radiotherapy has a distinct role in treating early cases of anal carcinoma. Tumors affecting half of the anal verge or less can be treated successfully by an interstitial implant. In more advanced cases carefully planned external irradiation is indicated prior to surgery. Although results are good, this method is not employed often because the number of suitable cases is limited.

SALIVARY GLAND TUMORS

Salivary gland tumors are characterized by their long natural history and frequent recurrences. They affect both the major salivary glands (parotid, submandibular, and sublingual) and the minor salivary glands. Since they occur in the region of the head and neck, indiscriminate therapeutic measures may result in more suffering than that caused by the original disease.

Pathological types

The most common types of pathological salivary gland tumors are shown in the following list:

Benign	Malignant
Pleomorphic adenoma (mixed parotid tumor)	Pleomorphic adenocarcinoma (malignant mixed parotid tumor)
	Adenoid cystic carcinoma (cylindroma)
	Adenocarcinoma
	Mucoepidermoid carcinomas
	Anaplastic carcinomas

Clinical picture

Usually there is a swelling, but rarely is there pain or nerve paralysis (such as in the facial nerve in parotid tumors), which is a sign of malignant infiltration.

The tumor *spread* is slow and localized. Malignant parotid tumors may involve the facial nerve or extend deeply to involve the faucial region (tonsils), lateral pharyngeal wall, or palate. Nerve involvement is especially common in cylindroma. *Lymphatic spread* is relatively late and primarily to the upper deep cervical and submandibular nodes. It occurs in about 25% of the cases. *Distant spread* to lungs and bones is rare. Patients can live for several years (some up to 5 years) despite the presence of pulmonary metastases.

Treatment policy

This depends on the pathological type as well as the extent of the lesion. Adequate excision of mixed parotid tumor (pleomorphic adenoma) by conservative parotidectomy sparing the facial nerve is sufficient to achieve cure. Alternatively, simple excision supplemented by radiotherapy yields the same results with perhaps less risk of operative facial injury.

Various combinations of aggressive radiotherapy and surgery are recommended for *malignant tumors.* When there is clinical evidence of malignant invasion (such as nerve paralysis) preoperative radiotherapy followed by surgical excision with supplementary radiotherapy to any residual disease seems to yield the best results. However, these cases are a minority. The majority of patients present with a tumor that proves to be malignant after histological examination of the surgical specimen. In this case, postoperative radiotherapy is recommended. Every attempt should be made to save the facial nerve (if uninvolved with disease) since radiotherapy is effective in sterilizing residual disease.

There is a definite place for *discriminate palliation* of bleeding, pain, and ulceration, usually by radiation, in advanced cases in view of the long natural history of the disease. Indeed indiscriminate use of surgery or radiotherapy in these cases may result not only in a high degree of morbidity but also substantial mortality. Radiotherapy technique consists of an external beam with a wedge distribution aiming for a dose of 5000 to 6000 rads in 5 to 6 weeks. Cervical nodes are treated only when involved.

Prognosis

With proper management no patient should die from pleomorphic adenoma and the percentage of local recurrence should be less than 5%.

Results of treatment of the malignant types, except for the low-grade mucoepidermoid tumors, are generally disappointing and about two thirds of the patients ultimately succumb to the disease.

MALIGNANT THYROID TUMORS

Malignant thyroid tumors form 1% of all the malignant tumors. Thyroid malignancies (follicular adenocarcinoma) represent the most important example of a functioning malignant tissue that is capable of retaining the parent-cell property of concentrating iodine and secreting thyroxin. Therefore, it lends itself to diagnosis and treatment by radioactive iodine (^{131}I). Thyroid malignancies occur most commonly in women. Although toxic goiter is not a *predisposing factor,* about 5% of nontoxic multinodular goiter contain malignant foci with increasing frequency (15%) in solitary nodules. Irradiation of thymus or tuberculous adenopathy in childhood predisposes to thyroid cancer early in life. Indeed 80% of children with thyroid cancer have a history of previous external irradiation. The main histological types (95%) are the differentiated carcinomas, including the papillary and follicular adenocarcinomas in addition to the anaplastic carcinomas. The differentiated carcinomas occur most commonly in the fourth and fifth decades of life, whereas the sixth and seventh decades represent the peak *age* incidence for the anaplastic ones.

Spread of these lesions varies according to the histology. Papillary adenocarcinoma spreads relatively early to cervical nodes, including the pretracheal and paratracheal nodes, which are usually slow growing. Locally, the disease is often multifocal in both thyroid lobes, but rarely does it extend beyond the thyroid capsule. Sometimes the disease presents with a lymph node metastasis in the cervical chain, whereas the primary is occult. Hematological spread is relatively rare, with lungs and bones being the most common sites. Anaplastic tumors on the other hand spread locally through the capsule to invade the trachea, esophagus, recurrent laryngeal nerve (causing cord paralysis), and sympathetic nerve (causing Horner's syndrome). Lymph node metastasis to the cervical chain and mediastinal nodes occurs relatively early, but grows rather fast, leading to superior mediastinal obstruction. Hematological spread may occur but is not reported widely, since the life-span of the patients is usually too short to allow for this.

Tracheal pressure, esophageal obstruction, laryngeal paralysis, and superior mediastinal obstruction are the most common *pathological complications.*

The presenting *clinical picture* varies according to the histological condition of the disease. Papillary and follicular adenocarcinoma usually presents with a thyroid nodule or a cervical node (metastasis). Anaplastic carcinoma on the other hand usually presents with pathological complications, especially tracheal pressure (dyspnea, stridor) and esophageal obstruction (dysphagia) or laryngeal paralysis (stridor, hoarseness of voice).

In addition to the usual *investigations* (see p. 87) the thyroid scan, which may reveal a cold nodule, is probably the most important diagnostic procedure. Thyroid cancer is rare in hyperfunctioning glandular tissue; so a nonfunctioning solitary nodule (cold nodule) must be suspect. Thyroid studies (to evaluate the thyroid function), skeletal survey, bone scan, and chest x-ray examination are among other important tests.

Total or subtotal thyroidectomy after exploration is usually the next step for establishment of a histological diagnosis and represents the first step of *treatment* at the same time. Biopsy per se is usually frowned upon except when the lesion is fixed. Even then, removal of as much of the local tumor (and its extension) as possible is recommended. The place of radiotherapy depends on the following three histological types (follicular adenocarcinoma, papillary adenocarcinoma, and anaplastic carcinoma).

Follicular adenocarcinoma. Since a follicular adenocarcinoma is the lesion most likely to concentrate iodine (in about 40% of cases) intravenous ^{131}I is used to irradiate any deposits. After ablation of the normal thyroid tissue (preferably by surgery, but it may be performed by a high dose of ^{131}I, about 100 mc.), a tracer dose of about 100 to 200 microcuries (μc.) of radioactive iodine is given intravenously and a subsequent whole-body scan may reveal the presence of metastases that are able to concentrate iodine. The tumor iodine uptake test is only possible in the absence of normal thyroid tissue, which has the ability to concentrate all available iodine. The tumor is then treated with periodic doses of ^{131}I about every 3 months. The dose depends on the amount of functioning malignant tissues, but 80 mc. is an average dose. In between doses the patient is kept on high doses of thyroxin (short of toxicity).

Nowadays the above management is limited to cases with metastases. A solitary nodule is treated by subtotal thyroidectomy followed by high doses of thyroxin. This treatment has the advantage of sparing parathyroid tissue.

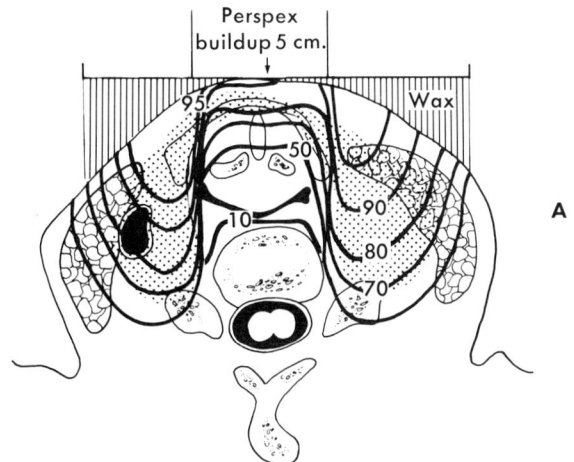

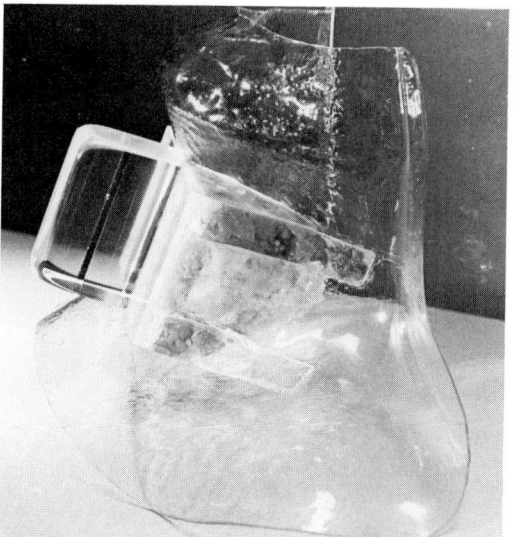

FIG. 9-10. **A,** Plan of treatment employing a 20 Mev. electron beam with central Perspex (methacrylic acid) buildup to avoid overirradiating the pharynx and spinal cord. Patient is treated in the cast shown, **B,** and the Perspex buildup is also shown.

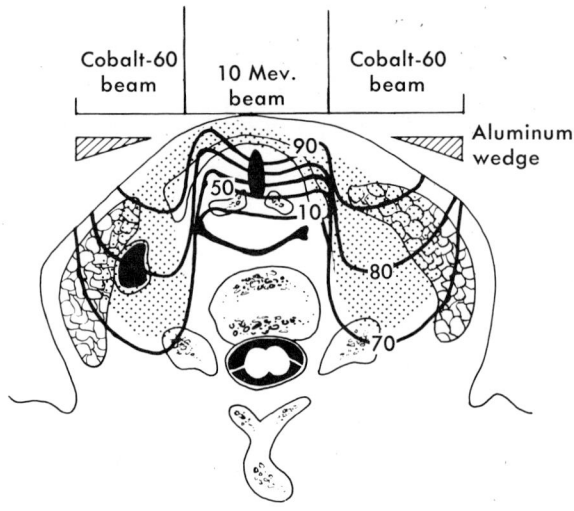

Fig. 9-11. Plan of treatment of carcinoma of thyroid, employing a cobalt-60 beam for lesion in both lobes and a 10 Mev. electron beam for the isthmus region.

Papillary adenocarcinoma. The same line of management is followed, but the percentage of functioning tumors is much smaller. Attention to complete surgical extirpation of the disease is necessary because of its multifocal nature. Such an approach followed by high-dose thyroxin yields very satisfactory survival rates.

Anaplastic carcinoma. After surgery, a postoperative course of radiotherapy is recommended. A plan designed to deliver the treatment is shown in Figs. 9-10 and 9-11. The dose aimed at is about 5000 rads in 5 weeks. The fields of treatment are usually large and may include the superior mediastinum.

Prognosis

The long-term results of the differentiated carcinomas, especially the localized forms, are excellent in that they approach the 90% mark particularly in younger patients. The results for anaplastic carcinomas are much poorer, with the 5-year survival rate being around 15%.

CHAPTER 10

BREAST MALIGNANCIES

Carcinoma of the breast is the most common malignancy and is the leading cause of death in American women, in whom it causes over 32,000 deaths yearly. The disease affects about 80 per 100,000 women and over 70,000 American women each year are newly diagnosed as having the disease. The peak *age* incidence is around 60 years. Only about 1% of all breast carcinomas occur in men.

Voluminous literature has been written about breast carcinoma and most known aspects have been discussed ad nauseum. In the following paragraphs we have summarized the most relevant facts. Breast carcinoma has been claimed to be commoner in women without children and related to age at first pregnancy (commoner in women first pregnant after 35 years of age), breast feeding (commoner in women who have not suckled), and hormonal irregularities (estrogen compounds especially estradiol are suspect) as *predisposing factors*, but the importance of these are subject to change as more statistics are accumulated. Trauma was also blamed by some authors and recently breast cancer has been linked to the presence of viruses in the milk (types B virus and C murine virus), but none of the above factors are beyond questioning at the moment.

Table 10-1 shows the different pathological types of breast malignancies. Breast carcinoma is by far the most common, especially infiltrating duct carcinoma (poorly differentiated adenocarcinoma).

Breast carcinoma is not uniform in its *spread;* some may grow and metastasize very slowly, and some grow and metastasize rapidly, whereas still others spread widely with minimal local growth. Present-day concepts underline the tumor-host interaction, which may determine the rate of growth and degree of metastasis.

The modified Tornberg classification is designed to demonstrate the relation between local growth and metastases and takes into account the grading of differentiation and degree of infiltration by lymphocytes and plasma cells (possible immune response).

Type 1 Nonmetastasizing: comedo carcinoma without stromal involvement

Type 2 Rarely metastasizing: mucinous or colloid carcinomas, medullary carcinoma with lymphocytic infiltration, and well-differentiated adenocarcinoma

Type 3 Moderately metastasizing: adenocarcinoma and intradductal carcinoma with stromal invasion

Type 4 Highly metastasizing: undifferentiated carcinoma and blood vessel invasion

Although local spread is usually the first to occur, occult breast carcinomas that present with nodal metastases are not unknown. The lesion usually starts in one of the breast quarters and for a time continues to be limited to that quarter before it eventually spreads to involve the skin and fungate through it or may infiltrate and fix to the pectoral muscle and chest wall eventually. The infiltration of the connective tissue produces contraction of the dermal papillae and of Cooper's ligaments, accompanied by lymphatic stasis, leading to the orange-peel appearance *(peau d'orange)*. Regional lymphatic spread is fairly common, with 30% of the cases presenting with lymph node metastasis. The site of the first nodal station depends on the site of the original disease; for example, lesions in the outer quadrants (commonest) spread first to axillary nodes with decreasing frequency of involvement from below upwards. When the axillary nodes are positive and the lesion is in the outer half of the breast, the parasternal (or internal mammary) nodes are involved in about 30% of cases and increase to more than 50% when the lesion is in the inner quadrants. The supraclavicular nodes may become involved subsequent to the presence of disease in the axilla. The lower and middle deep cervical nodes become involved less frequently.

Hematological spread is unpredictable; it may occur very late, on occasions after 20 years of disease, or very early. This is attributed, in part, to factors such as hormonal dependence or the presence or absence of the immune response. However, a lesion that presents with nodal metastases or that shows signs of rapid growth (such as inflammatory carcinoma) is more likely to disseminate early. Lungs, bones, adrenals, and the liver are the most common sites of metastasis, but no organ is exempt (such as the brain). The other breast and axilla are involved in about 15% of the cases depending on histologic types but the decision on whether this is metastatic or a new primary is often difficult, since such lesions do occur in about 6% of the cases.

Metastases account for the majority of *pathological complications* and are summarized as follows: pathological fractures (bone metastasis), anemia (bone marrow replacement by tumor or malignant depression of the marrow), suprarenal failure (suprarenal metastasis), pulmonary complications (malignant lymphangitic spread, pulmonary nodules, pleural effusion), and cerebral disorganization (brain metastasis) or malignant neuropathies. Metabolic abnormalities, such as increased serum calcium, is not uncommon in cases with extensive bone metastases.

Clinically, the most common presenting picture is a mass in the breast that on examination may reveal fixation to skin, muscle, or chest wall. The skin may be thickened (from lymphatic obstruction) and may show an "orange-peel" picture. Occasionally, the presenting picture may be an eczematoid lesion in a thickened skin (Pag-

TABLE 10-1. Pathological types of breast malignancies

Carcinoma
  Mammary ducts
    Noninfiltrating
      Papillary carcinoma
      Duct carcinoma
    Infiltrating
      Paget's disease
      Papillary carcinoma
      Comedo carcinoma
      Scirrhous carcinoma
        (adenocarcinoma with fibrosis)
      Medullary carcinoma
      Mucinous carcinoma
  Mammary lobules
    Noninfiltrating
      In situ
    Infiltrating
      Lobular adenocarcinoma
  Acute inflammatory carcinoma
Sarcoma

et's disease), which is always accompanied with an underlying duct carcinoma. Clinical examination should include examination of the ipsilateral axilla, other breast and axilla, and both supraclavicular and cervical regions to detect any nodal metastasis.

There are a number of different systems for the *clinical staging* of breast carcinoma. The following is suggested by the International Union Against Cancer:

T1	Less than 2 cm. no skin fixation
T2	2 to 5 cm. Skin infiltrated or ulcerated No pectoral fixation
T3	5 to 10 cm. Skin infiltrated or ulcerated Pectoral fixation
T4	More than 10 cm. Skin involvement not beyond breast Chest wall fixation
M0	No metastases
M1	Metastases including skin involvement beyond breast and contralateral nodes
N0	No nodes
N1	Axillary nodes movable
N1a	Not significant
N1b	Significant
N2	Axillary nodes fixed
N3	Supraclavicular nodes Edema of arm

The following four stage groupings are therefore designated by the TNM symbols:

Stage I	T1 N0 M0 T2 N0 M0
Stage II	T1 N1 M0 T2 N1 M0
Stage III	T1 N2 or N3 M0 T2 N2 or N3 M0 T3 N0, N1, N2, or N3 M0 T4 N0, N1, N2, or N3 M0
Stage IV	Any combination of T and N symbols including M1

Since the Columbia classification was the first to show the relevance of clinical staging to treatment policy and prognosis, it is important to be aware of its outline:

Stage A 1. No clinically involved axillary nodes
2. No grave signs like those enumerated in stage C
Stage B 1. Clinically involved axillary nodes less than 2.5 cm.
2. No grave signs like those in stage C
Stage C Any one of five grave signs
1. Edema of skin (less than one third of skin involved)
2. Ulceration of skin
3. Fixation to chest wall
4. Axillary nodes greater than 2.5 cm.
5. Fixed axillary nodes to surrounding tissues
Stage D All more advanced cases

Stages A and B were deemed amenable to radical mastectomy, whereas stages C and D were not.

Investigations include chest x-ray examination, mammography (to both breasts), skeletal survey, a liver scan, and a bone scan. The last is especially indicated if there are symptoms suggestive of bony metastasis in the presence of negative diagnostic roentgenograms. Necessary blood chemistry includes serum calcium and alkaline phosphatase (raised in bone metastasis). Biopsy for histological diagnosis is the single most important test to establish diagnosis.

The *treatment* of operable breast carcinoma has lead to more controversy than the treatment of almost all the other malignancies combined. The role of radiotherapy and surgery is still unresolved and has resulted in a variety of proposed treatment procedures, ranging from simple excision of the tumor (lumpectomy) to superradical mastectomy. The results of cooperative studies including prospective controlled clinical trials have not resolved therapeutic differences and no one procedure currently used is universally regarded as satisfactory. The role of chemotherapy in the treatment of operable breast cancer is under active investigation, and early results indicate that it may be beneficial. Table 10-2 lists the available policies that combine surgery with radiotherapy.

There is less controversy regarding the treatment of advanced breast cancer. Radical surgery is inapplicable because the disease has spread beyond the limits of resec-

110 *Clinical radiation oncology*

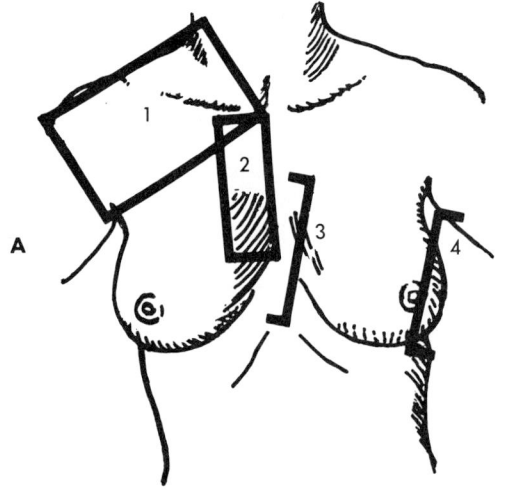

Fig. 10-1. **A**, Technique of postoperative treatment in carcinoma of the breast. *1*, Supraclavicular field. *2*, Parasternal field. *3* and *4*, Lateral tangential fields. **B**, Check film for a lateral tangential field for treatment of a breast carcinoma.

TABLE 10-2. Operable breast cancer

Surgery	Radiotherapy with surgery
1. Simple excision (tumorectomy, lumpectomy)—removal of malignant focus from breast	1. Radiation directed to the breast, axilla, and internal mammary and supraclavicular nodes
2. Simple mastectomy (total mastectomy)—removal of breast only	2. Radiation to chest wall, axilla, and internal mammary and supraclavicular nodes
3. Modified radical mastectomy (removal of breast, pectoralis minor, and axillary nodes)—the pectoralis major is left intact	3. Same as (2)
4. Radical mastectomy (removal breast, pectoralis major and minor muscles, and axillary lymph nodes)	4. Radiation to only internal mammary and supraclavicular nodes (including axillary apex) if breast lesion is in the inner quadrants or subareolar area or if axillary nodes are positive. The chest wall is irradiated if 20% or more of the axillary nodes are malignant in order to reduce local recurrence
5. Superradical mastectomy (radical mastectomy plus internal mammary node dissection)	5. Seldom used
6. Extended radical mastectomy (superradical mastectomy plus supraclavicular node dissection, or, in another variety, removal of mediastinal nodes)	6. Seldom used

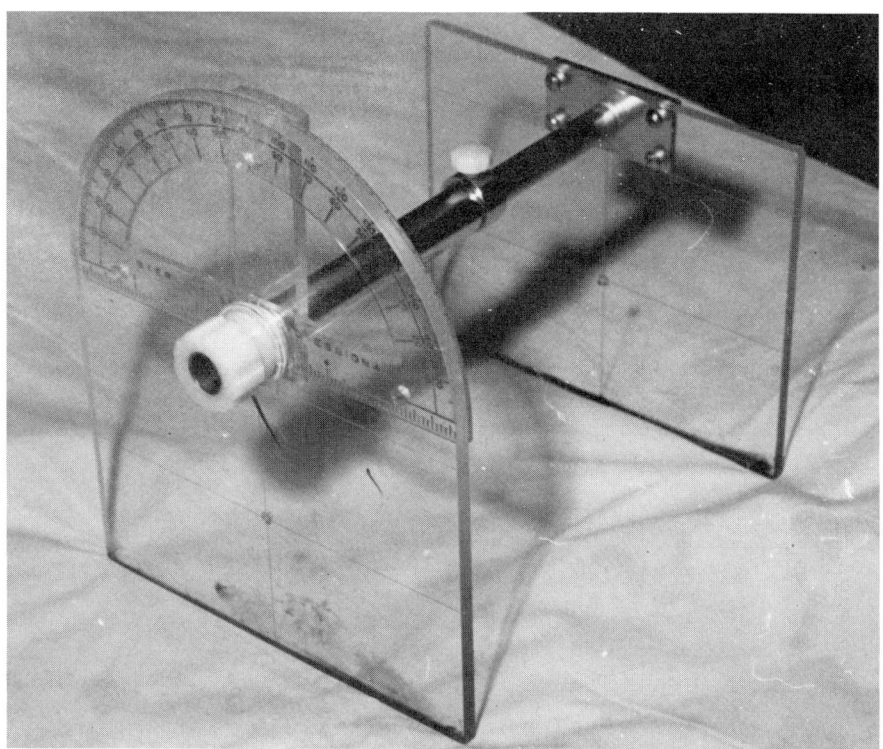

Fig. 10-2. Breast bridge.

tion. The aim of treatment is to control local and regional disease either by limited "cleansing" simple mastectomy, or radiotherapy, or both. It is preferable to remove large masses surgically prior to radiotherapy. However, if surgery is not feasible, protracted radiation may control the disease successfully.

Subsequent management depends on the spread and extent of the disease. Chemotherapeutic agents, hormonal therapy, and hormonal ablation procedures (oophorectomy, irradiation of both ovaries, adrenalectomy) are used in various combinations, depending on the particular problem at hand.

In *techniques of radiotherapy*, we realize that there are several used, but the one described in Fig. 10-1 is simple, adequate, and practical. It shows the field arrangements for the treatment of the draining nodes (axillary, supraclavicular, and parasternal). Fig. 10-2 shows a breast bridge used to facilitate the setup for treatment of the breast or chest wall by two tangential fields. In the post–radical mastectomy operation (where the axillary nodes are dissected), the technique is slightly modified to limit the treatment to the apical axillary nodes, supraclavicular nodes, and parasternal nodes. The radiation used is usually a gamma beam or a supervoltage beam. The dose aimed at varies according to the objective. If the disease is subclinical (or presumed to be so), the dose is 4500 to 5000 rads in 5 weeks, whereas if it is gross, the dose is higher, 6000 to 7000 rads in 6 weeks. This dose could be supplemented either by a small field or a radium implant for an additional 1000 to 2000 rads.

Complications of such treatment are rather limited; skin reaction (erythema and dry or moist desquamation) may occur toward the end of treatment, but its management is simple (see p. 57). Dysphagia may occur as a result of irradiation of a segment of the esophagus. The management of this reaction is described on p. 59. Late reaction such as skin atrophy, telangiectasia, and pulmonary fibrosis should be minimal (if ever) with careful execution of the above plan.

The breast, or chest wall, is usually treated by two tangential fields, with use of a bolus during the first half of the treatment. Care must be taken not to irradiate a large section of the lungs.

The prognosis depends mainly on the stage of the disease at presentation—the higher the stage, the worse the prognosis. The 5-year survival rate is 75%, 50%, 30%, and 15%, for stages I to IV, respectively. Factors that indicate poor prognosis other than clinical staging are high-grade malignancy, inflammatory carcinoma, presence of four or more positive nodes in a surgical specimen, involvement of the nipple by a tumor, and absence of signs of immune response. In addition, men with mammary cancer have a worse prognosis than do women.

The 5-year survival figures are not a true enough indicator of cure, since a majority of these patients are rather young and the disease may recur after longer intervals. The 10-year survival figures in stages I and II are 65% and 22%, respectively.

CHAPTER 11

FEMALE GENITAL SYSTEM

Tumors of the female genital system are second only to those of the breast in their frequency. They affect about 70 of every 100,000 women in the United States.

The female genital system is formed of *four anatomical zones,* which are distinctive from each other both in their anatomical and physiological relationships and the malignant lesions that afflict them. Almost all tumors of the female genital system are characterized by their ability for spreading to both sides of the body.

Zone A consists of the vulva and the lower part of the vagina. Since the tissues are epithelial, their common tumors are epidermoid carcinomas, which spread mainly by local invasion and lymphatic dissemination to the inguinal and femoral nodes.

Zone B, composed of the cervix (and cervical canal) and the upper part of the vagina is lined by stratified squamous epithelium (being the origin of squamous cell carcinoma), in addition to numerous glandular follicles (adenocarcinomas) in the cervical canal. The main method of spread is by direct invasion and lymphatic metastases.

Zone C consists of the uterus and tubes. The endometrium lining the uterus is very active glandular tissue that undergoes cyclical changes during menstruation. The lining epithelium of the fallopian tubes is the ciliated columnar type. Consequently, the common malignant lesions are adenocarcinomas. Since lymphatics are rather scanty and found mainly in the muscle and serous layers, spread by this route is both relatively rare and late. Although choriocarcinomas occur in the uterus, they originate in the placental tissue of a fetus and so may be considered foreign to the uterus itself.

Zone D is formed of the ovaries, which possess a complicated and protean structure and so give rise to multiple tumor types. The ovary is a peritoneal structure and the main method of spread of its tumors is by peritoneal seeding, beside local and nodal spread.

VULVA AND LOWER VAGINA

Malignant tumors of the vulva are the second rarest of all the female genital system lesions (about 4%). They commonly occur in the elderly (in the seventh decade). Senile keratitis, leukoplakia, kraurosis, and diabetic vulvitis may play a *predisposing role*. Squamous cell carcinomas are the commonest *pathological* type followed by malignant melanoma, but any skin malignancy may occur, including adenocarcinomas arising from Bartholin's gland. The lesion is usually a malignant ulcer by the time it presents for treatment. *Spread* of vulvar lesions is mainly by direct invasion inward from a labium majus to a labium minus and laterally from one labium to the other of the same type. Lymphatic spread is fairly common and relatively early, with the inguinal nodes being the first site affected. Both sides (nodes) are prone to be involved even if the lesion is unilateral. Later spread to femoral and iliac nodes may occur. Lymphatic obstruction and edema is the main *pathological complication,* occurring especially in late cases, and denotes spread to iliac nodes. Pain from involvement of nerves is another complication.

Lymphangiography is a method of *investigation* that may succeed in demonstrating the extent of nodal involvement although the studies conducted so far have met with limited success.

The main method of *treatment* is radical vulvectomy where both the vulva and the vagina are excised and the nodes are dissected. The role of *radiotherapy,* which continues to be controversial, is summarized as follows:
1. Curative to early unilateral small lesions. The technique of choice would be an interstitial implant using radium or better still an afterloading technique using radioactive iridium seeds or tantalum wires. The dose aimed at should be about 6000 to 6500 rads. In extensive lesions external irradiation is used to reduce the tumor size prior to the implant.
2. Preoperative or postoperative treatment to the inguinal nodes aiming at improving the results of treatment by reduction of local recurrences.
3. Palliative radiotherapy directed to inguinal nodes when they are fixed or so extensive that cure is unattainable. This may achieve tumor regression as well as prevent fungation and eliminate pain. The technique of choice would be by external irradiation with a highly penetrating beam (gamma beam or supervoltage x rays). The dose aimed at is 5000 rads in about 5 weeks.

Tolerance and complications of treatment

The region of the vulva and perineum is claimed to have a low tolerance to radiation because of the excessive moisture, warmth, and usual soiling of the skin. An excessive skin reaction used to be a common sequence, especially with the employment of conventional beams or even with supervoltage beams in the presence of multiple creases (which tend to nullify the skin-sparing effect). However, the judicial choice of the beam, the proper employment of wedges, a reduced daily dose fraction, and an appropriate small volume would enable the radiotherapist to deliver an effective treatment without an undue degree of tissue damage.

Prognosis

Early lesions less than 3 cm. in diameter have a 5-year survival rate of about 70%, but late lesions with nodal spread have a very poor outlook (10% 5-year survival).

CERVIX

Carcinoma of the cervix is the most common malignancy of the female genital system (50%). It is most common in the fourth and fifth decades of life.

The disease is particularly rare among Jews and relatively rare in Muslims. This is attributed to the practice of circumcision among both these groups. The smegma in the semen of the uncircumcised male has been blamed as a *predisposing factor*. This is also supported by the fact that cervical carcinoma is more rare in women using a diaphragm as a contraceptive, compared to those using other methods. Increasing degree of parity as well as lower socioeconomic conditions are associated with increased incidence of the disease.

The most common *pathological type* of cervical carcinoma is squamous cell carcinoma (over 90%), followed by adenocarcinoma. Cervical carcinoma *spreads* mainly by local extension to involve the vaginal fornices, lower vagina, both parametria, bladder, and rectum. *Lymphatic* involvement is fairly common even in the earlier stages of the disease. When the disease is limited to the cervix, nodal metastases may amount to 15% to 20% of the cases, with increasing percentage in later stages of the disease (up to 60% in stage III). Bloodborne metastases are relatively rare (5%), but they have been encountered with increasing frequency recently as local treatment becomes more effective and patients with advanced stages of the disease live longer.

As the spread of cervical cancer dictates the treatment plan and influences prognosis, *clinical staging* becomes extremely important. The following system of international staging has been evolved:

Stage 0	Preinvasive disease (Smear test is positive and biopsy shows the disease to be noninvasive); may be called carcinoma in situ
Stage I	Disease limited to the cervix
Stage II	Disease involving vagina (not more than upper third), or parametrium (but not fixed to pelvic walls), or both
Stage III	Disease fixed to pelvic walls, or the lower third of the vagina, or both
Stage IV	Disease involving bladder or rectum

Note that this staging is limited to the tumor only (T). It is not related to nodes (N) or metastases (M). Furthermore stages II and III are subdivided into A and B according to the extent of the spread, as follows:

Stage IIA	Vaginal involvement only
Stage IIB	Parametrial involvement
Stage IIIA	Disease limited to one side or lower third of vagina
Stage IIIB	Disease spread to both sides

Ureteral involvement (mainly at the uterovesical junction in the root of the parametrium), with secondary hydronephrosis and uremia, is the most important *pathological complication*. Pain from neural involvement is another feature of advanced local disease and often exhibits a sciatic distribution (involvement of lumbosacral plexus). Edema of the lower limbs may result from extensive lymphatic involvement and obstruction.

Vaginal bleeding is the most common *symptom* of cervical carcinoma. Sometimes occurring in the early stages is pain caused by obstruction of the cervical opening with subsequent infection and pyometra (leading to suprapubic pain). An ulcerating lesion is the usual finding at examination.

Examination under anesthesia is the most important *investigation* in the clinical staging of the disease. Cystoscopy, intravenous pyelography, barium enema, and sigmoidoscopy are other necessary tests. Lymphangiography is used to a lesser extent.

The *treatment* of cervical carcinoma depends mainly on the stage of the disease and is predominantly by radiation therapy apart from stage 0, wherein hysterectomy produces excellent results (95% 5-year survival rate).

Radiation therapy is usually applied by use of external irradiation and intracavitary insertion (of radium or cesium) in various combinations and sequences depending on the stage of the disease. There is no unanimous agreement about the combination; however external irradiation is emphasized in more advanced or higher stage disease. This accomplishes a reduction of the tumor bulk and sterilization of disease in the nodal regions. Consequently radium application becomes more efficient. The following summary represents a good working arrangement:

Stage I	Two radium insertions followed by external irradiation to parametrium (4000 rads in 4 weeks). Bulky disease may require prior external irradiation in order to make dose distribution from the radium application acceptable.
Stage IIa	External irradiation (2000 rads) to whole pelvis plus two radium insertions plus external irradiation (2000 to 3000 rads) to the parametrium (Fig. 11-1).
Stage IIb	External irradiation (4000 rads in 4 weeks) to whole pelvis (Fig. 11-2)

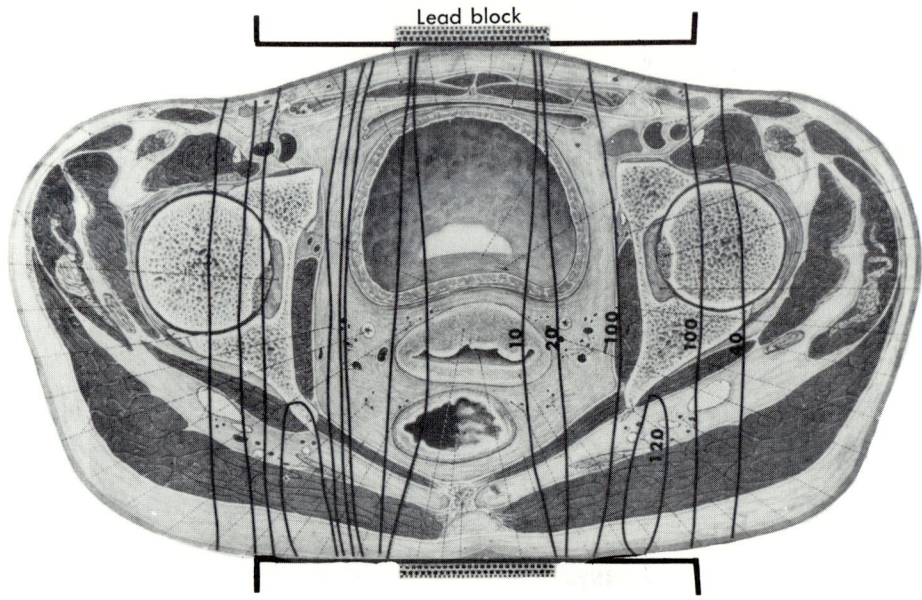

Fig. 11-1. Plan of treatment of both parametria after radium insertion. Notice falloff of dose caused by lead block.

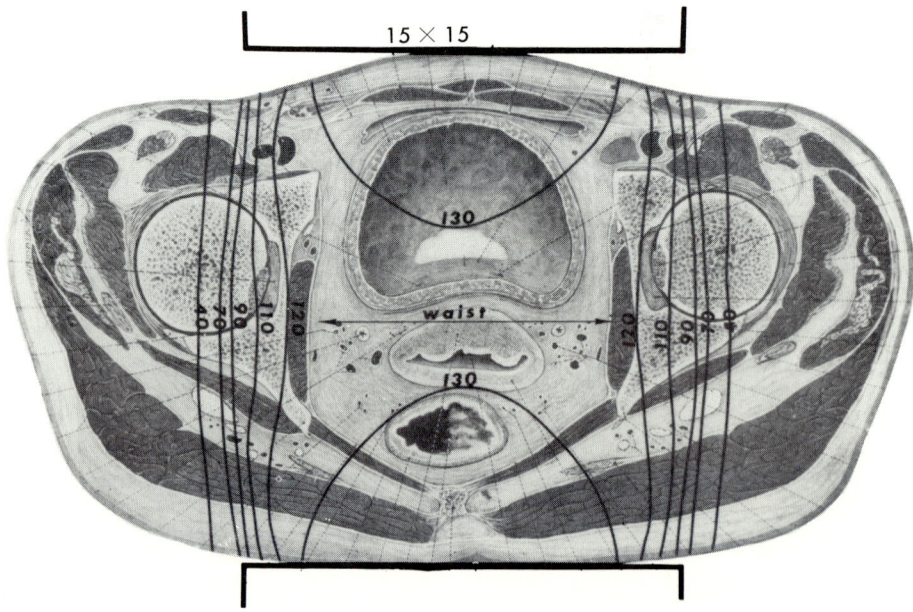

Fig. 11-2. Plan of treatment of whole pelvis using two opposed fields.

plus two radium insertions. Further irradiation will depend on the extent of the disease and the dosage calculated to various structures and whether subsequent surgery is contemplated (extrafascial hysterectomy).

Stage III   External irradiation to whole pelvis (about 6000 rads in 6 weeks). Further management will depend on the response of the disease.

Stage IV   External irradiation given depends on the extent of the lesion in each case.

Some patients may stand to benefit from subsequent pelvic evisceration.

Technique of radiotherapy

External irradiation. The beam used should have a high penetrating quality, such as a ^{60}Co beam with a sufficiently long source-to-skin distance (about 80 cm.) or a supervoltage x-ray beam. Fields applied usually include the whole pelvis, lower para-aortic, and common iliac nodes. A central lead block of 4 to 5 cm. in width and appropriate thickness is used to protect the rectum and bladder during parametrial irradiation (Fig. 11-1).

Intracavitary radium. Several applicators have been designed for inserting radium into the uterus and vaginal vault. The Manchester, Paris, Stockholm, Ernst, and Fletcher are only a few examples. The Fletcher afterloading applicators are gaining popularity in this country (Fig. 11-3). They are basically composed of two ovoid colpostats and a uterine tandem made of stainless steel. The applicators are designed in such a way that radium can be inserted through them after the operation and after checking their position by x-ray film. This allows more time and thought to the amount of radium to be used and better designing of the dosage. Moreover, exposure to technicians and doctors is kept to a minimal level. Fig. 11-4 shows the distribution of the isodose curves in such an insertion. The dose aimed at varies from one case to the other, but generally each insertion lasts for 48 to 72 hours. Historically dose calculations were determined at two arbitrary points termed "point A" and "point B" (see glossary). Doses to the rectum and bladder can also be calculated as well as measured directly.

Complications of treatment

The fact that two systems for delivering radiation (external beam and intracavitary radium) are generally used in cervical lesions, predispose to overdosage (or underdosage) and subsequent complications.

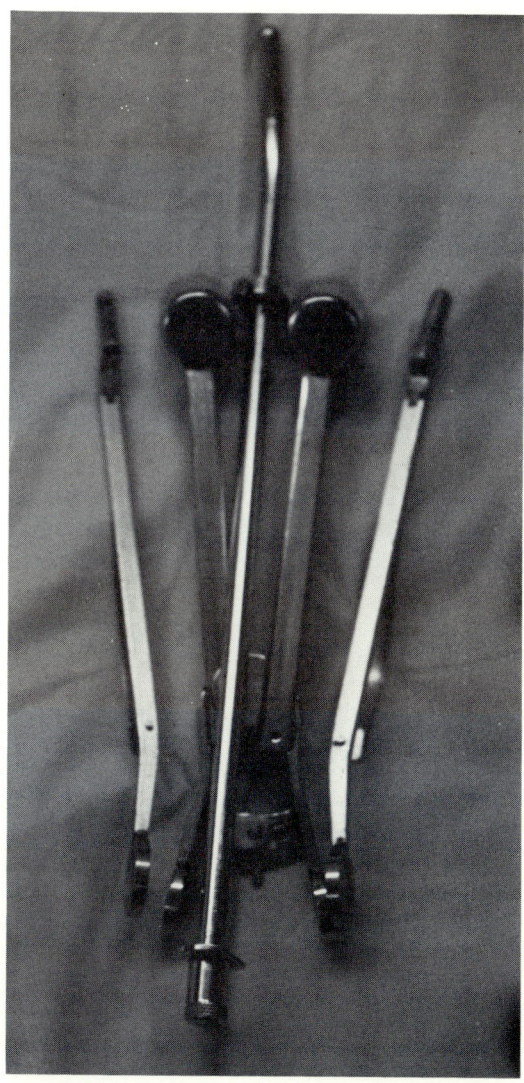

FIG. 11-3. Applicators for insertion of radium into uterus. (Developed by G. Fletcher and H. Suit, M. A. Anderson Hospital.)

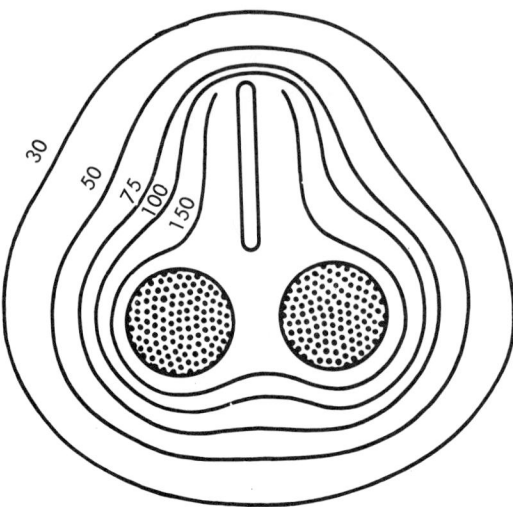

FIG. 11-4. Isodose curves of a radium insertion.

The early side effects of treatment may vary from mild to severe diarrhea, and abdominal cramps. Urinary symptoms (dysurea and greater frequency) may occur but are less common. General constitutional disturbances (so-called radiation sickness) are rarely encountered and almost only in cases where external irradiation was delivered to the whole pelvis in large doses. Late vaginal adhesions may be bothersome. Diarrhea usually responds to simple measures like kaopectate and, if more severe, opiates or opiate-like drugs (such as diphenoxylate [Lomotil] tablets). On occasions, it may be advisable to suspend the treatment for a few days. Urinary symptoms are relieved by mild antiseptics (such as phenazopyridine HCl [Pyridium] tablets) and bladder antispasmodics (such as propantheline bromide [Pro-Banthine] tablets).

Late complications of treatment are more serious, though much less common. Intestinal obstruction, ulceration, or perforation may affect the sigmoid colon predominantly. Vesicovaginal or rectovaginal fistulas can occur in the more advanced stages. However, fistulas may occur through persistent disease in a good number of these cases and thorough investigations must be carried out before accepting this as a complication of treatment. In cases where the bladder was heavily irradiated, subsequent atrophy of the mucosa and telangiectasia may lead to hematuria. The treatment of most of these late complications may necessitate a surgical procedure (for fistula repair or intestinal obstruction). Postoperative morbidity after these surgically procedures is higher than in cases where no radiation was given.

The *prognosis* of cervical carcinomas has changed to a much happier picture in recent years. Cytological screening tests help to bring patients to treatment at an earlier stage of the disease. The availability of more penetrating beams of radiation has enabled the radiotherapist to deliver a higher dose with more accuracy. The 5-year survival rate is strictly related to the stage of the disease at presentation. In stage I about 90% of patients treated are alive and well after 5 years. In stage II, the figure drops to about 75%. In stage III, it is about 45%. The results in stage IV are still very poor (about 14%).

UTERUS

Endometrial carcinoma of the uterus is the second most common malignancy of the female gential system after that of the cervix (17 women in 100,000 population compared to 44 in 100,000). Although several forms of malignant lesions affect the uterus, adenocarcinoma is the most frequent (90%). Postmenopausal women in the sixth decade of life are those most susceptible.

The tumor may be related to long continued, cyclic stimulation of the endometrium by estrogen (and possibly progesterone) usually of ovarian origin.

The lesion *spreads* mainly by local invasion to the muscle layer as well as the serous coat. The tumor usually starts in the fundus of the uterus, but eventually it extends inferiorly to the lower uterine segment and cervical canal. Involvement of the latter structure changes the natural history of the tumor because it then tends to follow the lines of spread of cervical lesions (with lymphatic involvement). Endometrial carcinoma tends to spread to lymphatics late in the natural history of the disease, and in 75% of the cases the tumor is clinically confined to the uterus at the time of diagnosis. Bloodborne metastases are rarer still. Sometimes cells displaced from the tumor spread to the ovary, leading to secondary growth (4%).

The poorly differentiated type of endometrial carcinoma displays a higher incidence of local spread, as well as increased nodal and vaginal metastases giving rise to the worst prognosis.

Clinical staging of endometrial carcinoma is relatively recent and not widely accepted yet (as in the case of carcinoma of the cervix). The classification summarized here is that adopted by the International Federation of Gynecology and Obstetrics:

Stage 0   Preinvasive carcinoma, carcinoma in situ.
Stage I   Carcinoma is strictly confined to the corpus uteri.
Stage II Carcinoma has involved corpus uteri and cervix.
Stage III Carcinoma has extended outside the uterus but not outside the true pelvis.
Stage IVa Carcinoma has extended outside the true pelvis, or involved the bladder or rectum.
Stage IVb Any tumor as previously staged in combination with clinical or radiographic evidence of metastases outside the pelvis.

Although postmenopausal bleeding is the cardinal *symptom* of endometrial carcinoma, other symptoms such as suprapubic pain (in case of obstruction and pyometra) or feeling of pressure on rectum are not unknown.

Investigations are similar to the ones used in cervical carcinoma. However fractional curettage is of utmost important because it is the most important method of diagnosing involvement of the cervical canal.

Treatment depends on the stage of spread of the disease. A lesion that has involved the endocervix or the cervical canal is treated along the same lines as a carcinoma of the cervix. Otherwise, surgery (panhysterectomy) is the method of treatment most commonly used.

Radiotherapy plays a very important role both as complementary to surgery and as the definitive treatment. There is no general agreement about the method of applying radiotherapy (whether by external irradiation or intracavitary radium) or its timing when combined with surgery (preoperative or postoperative).

Preoperative intracavitary radium insertion is the most commonly used method, but many centers are using external irradiation for this purpose. This is usually followed by hysterectomy after a waiting period of 3 to 6 weeks. Results claimed after such treatment are highly satsifactory and complications of treatment are minimal. However, some authors claim that postoperative external irradiation is equally effective and is especially indicated in anaplastic lesions, lesions involving the myometrium, or those with nodal metastases. There is general agreement that radiation reduces the incidence of vaginal metastases.

The technique of external irradiation is very similar to that of cervical carcinoma with the aim of treating the whole pelvis (15×15 cm. size fields) up to a dose of about 4000 to 5000 rads in 4 to 5 weeks. Intracavitary radiation can be applied by use of the Fletcher applicators or the Heyman packing technique (Fig. 11-5). The latter technique (evolved by the Swedish pioneer Heyman) depends on the packing of the uterus with radium tubes (about 100 mg. of radium) in addition to two ovoids in the vaginal vault (10 mg. in each fornix). The system is left for about 16 to 18 hours.

If radiotherapy is the definitive treatment, the dose should be carried to higher or curative levels. This is especially indicated if the patient is a bad surgical risk or refuses the operation (these patients are usually obese and frequently suffer from hypertension and diabetes). Progestins

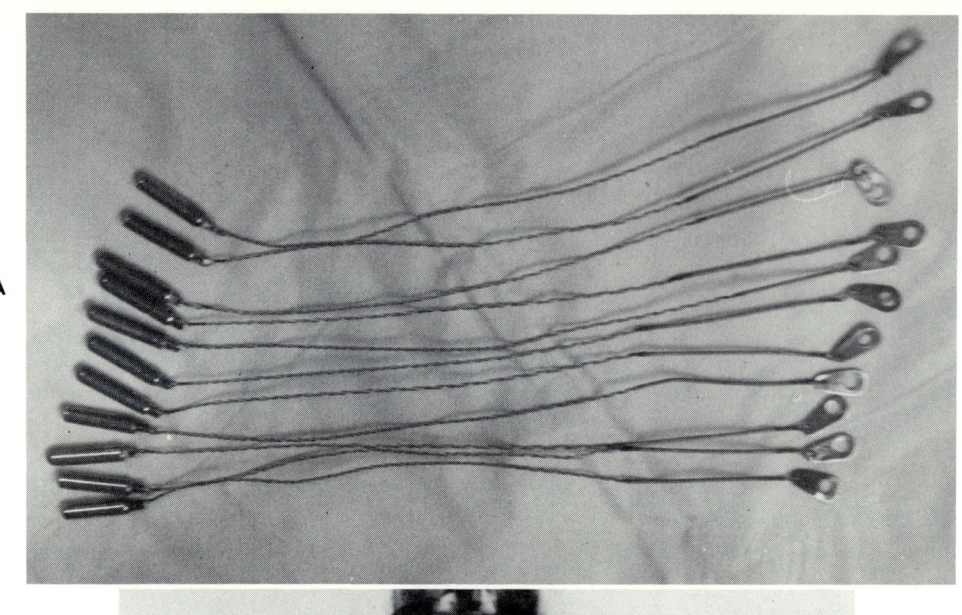

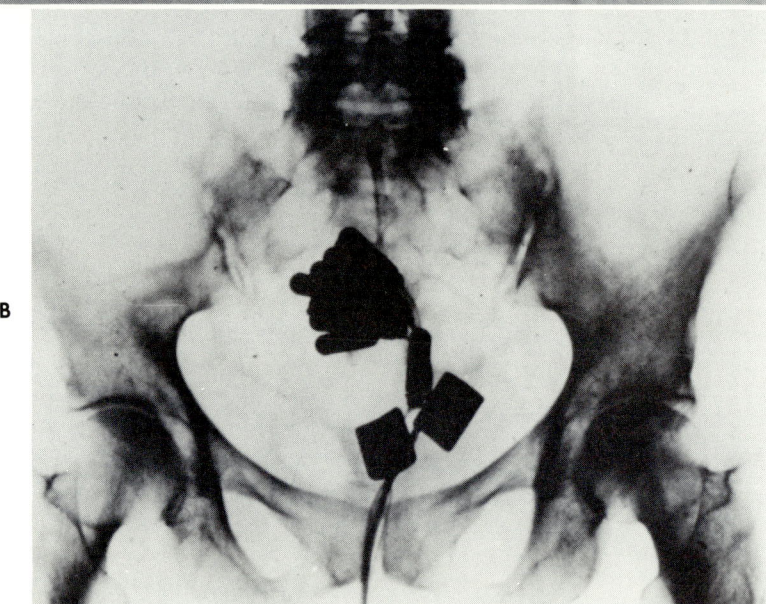

Fig. 11-5. **A,** Heyman applicators. **B,** Roentgenogram of pelvis area with Heyman applicators in place.

have been used in the treatment of disseminated endometrial adenocarcinoma with some success. Several dramatic reports of the disappearance of lung metastases exist.

The prognosis of endometrial carcinoma is generally more favorable than carcinoma of the cervix. The 5-year survival figure is about 90%. Myometrial involvement reduces the results to 70%. Cervical involvement reduces the figure further to 50%, whereas anaplastic tumors have a 40% survival rate. Cases with distant pelvic or general metastasis have a 5-year survival rate of 10%.

OVARY

Ovarian malignancies constitute the third most frequent gynecological cancer, with over 10,000 annual deaths. It is the fourth leading cause of death after breast, large bowel, and cervix malignancies.

The ovary is a complex structure and consists of various types of cells, which gives rise to several types of malignant tumors. The surface of the ovary is covered with a layer of cubical cells called the "germinal epithelium." After puberty the ovary has a thick cortex, which contains the ovarian follicles and corpora lutea, and surrounds a richly vascular medulla. During prenatal life the stroma of the cortex contains small groups of interstitial cells, but after puberty these cells are only present in the theca of atretic ovarian follicles. With this complex structure in mind, one can easily understand the following outline of *histological types:*

1. Gonadal stroma
   Malignant granulotheca cell tumor
   Malignant form of arrhenoblastoma (a musculizing tumor)
2. Germ cell tumors
   Pure germ cell type ... Dysgerminoma 5%
   Extraembryonic ...... Choriocarcinoma
   Embryonic.......... Malignant teratoma and teratocarcinomas
3. Germinal epithelium
   Cystoadenocarcinoma
     Mucous
     Serous
   Solid carcinoma
4. Metastatic tumors

The most common type is the cystadenocarcinoma (both serous and mucinous) on which our discussion concentrates. Since dysgerminoma has many characteristics relevant to radiotherapeutic management, we will also discuss it in some detail. Women in the fifth and sixth decades of life are the ones most commonly affected except in the case of dysgerminoma, which is most common in the second and third decades of life. Dysgerminoma may occur rarely in children.

Ovarian carcinomas *spread* mainly by local invasion and result in fixation of the ovary to the surrounding structures. Peritoneal spread by seedings is common and occurs early during the natural history of the disease. Such a spread affects the other ovary, omentum, and pouch of Douglas, but no peritoneal recess or fold is immune. Bloodborne metastases are next in frequency. Liver and splanchnic organs are the most common sites of metastases. Lymph node metastases occur relatively late in the natural history of the disease, except for dysgerminoma, which spreads early and mainly by lymphatic involvement.

The most important *pathological complications,* such as ascites, intestinal obstruction, and rarely ureteral obstruction (and hydronephrosis), are linked to the peritoneal spread.

Patients usually *present* with an abdominal swelling, ascites, or abdominal distention (from incomplete intestinal obstruction). A rapid increase in the skirt size of a woman 40 years of age is always suspicious and must be investigated carefully. Disturbances in the menstrual cycle is another presenting picture.

Clinical staging as adopted by the International Federation of Gynecology and Obstetrics is summarized as follows:

Stage I	Growth limited to the ovaries
Stage Ia	One ovary
Stage Ib	Both ovaries
Stage Ic	Ovary and ascites
Stage II	Growth involving one or both ovaries with pelvic extension.
Stage IIa	Extension to uterus or tubes, or both
Stage IIb	Extension to other pelvic tissues
Stage III	Growth involving one or both ovaries with widespread intraperitoneal metastases
Stage IV	Growth involving one or both ovaries with distant metastases outside the peritoneal cavity

Examination under anesthesia may reveal an ovarian mass and other *investigations,* such as intravenous pyelogram, barium enema, and chest x-ray film, may show the extent of the disease, but *laparotomy* is the only sure method for obtaining a pathological diagnosis.

Treatment of ovarian carcinomas is by surgical removal (oophorectomy and hysterectomy), but more often than not the disease is beyond complete surgical removal. Provided that there is no evidence of bloodborne metastases, postoperative radiotherapy is recommended. Chemotherapy is the main method of treatment in the presence of widespread bloodborne disease. Its place when the disease is still limited is debatable, but many authors claim that there is a beneficial effect. In the treatment of advanced carcinoma the sequential application of the three modalities may result in a significant increase in survivals.

The technique of radiotherapy will depend on the extent of the disease (pelvic or total abdomen). Deeply penetrating beams are necessary (supervoltage x-ray beam or gamma beam with a long SSD). The dosage aimed at is usually within about 5000 rads in 5 weeks to the pelvis and 3000 in 4 to 5 weeks to the total abdomen.

Effusion (which occurs in over three fourths of the patients) can be treated effectively by instillation of radioactive gold or phosphorus. External irradiation may be used effectively on occasions.

Prognosis depends largely on the stage (or extent) of the disease, the degree of differentiation of the tumor, and the histological type. However, there is always a certain element of unpredictability. The 5-year survival figure of stage I cases is about 65%; that of stage II is about 50%; in stage III, 35%; and in stage IV, 5%. The main cause of death is cachexia or intestinal obstruction caused by abdominal carcinomatosis.

Dysgerminoma

The variant of ovarian tumors called dysgerminoma is relatively rare (4% of ovarian tumors) and represents the female counterpart of seminoma. It commonly affects young patients in the second and third decades. The tumor *spreads* characteristically to lymph nodes and the peritoneum, but it may continue to be limited to the ovary for some time. The tumor is sometimes associated with hermaphroditism and pseudohermaphroditism. It may also be associated with other highly malignant tumors like choriocarcinoma. The disease is characterized by its high radiosensitivity, and so it stands unique from other ovarian tumors.

Treatment is summarized in surgical excision (salpingo-oophorectomy) followed by radiotherapy, which should include the para-aortic lymph nodes if their involvement by the disease is suspect. The technique is rather similar to that used in treatment of seminoma (see p. 126).

Prognosis depends on the extent of the disease, being excellent (95% 5-year survival rate) if it is limited to the ovary, but being rather poor (33% 5-year survival rate) if the disease had metastasized.

CHAPTER 12

MALE GENITAL SYSTEM

Malignancies of the male genital system originate commonly in one of three organs —penis, testis, and prostate gland (Fig. 12-1). These three organs are different from each other in structure, and so their lesions differ. Penile malignancies are usually of skin origin, those of the testis arise mostly from the germinal epithelium, and the prostatic lesions are almost exclusively adenocarcinomas arising from the glandular tissue.

PENIS

Malignant tumors of the penis are usually of skin origin and arise mainly in the frenum and prepuce (Fig. 12-1) and to a lesser extent in the glans and coronal sulcus. These lesions may occur at any age, but the sixth decade of life is the most common. The disease represents 0.3% to 0.5% of all cancers and is almost unknown in Jews and very rare in Muslims (because of circumcision). However, it is more common in Negroes (four times) in this country. Lack of hygiene, which may be associated with the presence of a tight prepuce (phimosis), has been blamed as a *predisposing factor*. Squamous cell carcinomas (well to moderately differentiated) are the most common malignancies, but basal cell carcinomas and malignant melanomas are not unknown. The lesions, which start usually in the prepuce or frenum, *spread* by local invasion of the penile corpora leading to its fixation and sometimes pain. The urethra may be involved if the disease is allowed to expand unchecked. Lymphatic spread to the bilateral inguinal nodes is fairly common (except in pure basal cell carcinomas) occurring in about 50% of the cases. The lesion usually presents *clinically* as an ulcer and requires biopsy for verification. The apparent similarity between this lesion and some venereal ulcers may be a cause of delay of diagnosis in some patients.

Treatment would depend on the extent of the disease. If the penile lesion is limited to skin (without involvement of the corpora), it can be treated successfully with irradiation (after circumcision or splitting of the prepuce), thus saving the penis and avoiding the psychic trauma of penile amputation. Furthermore sexual function may be maintained. Consequently, surgery can be reserved for radiation failures. Involvement of the corpora is usually an indication for surgery (amputation of the organ) although some cases may be treated by radiation, especially if the patient refuses operation or is a bad risk. Early involved

124 Clinical radiation oncology

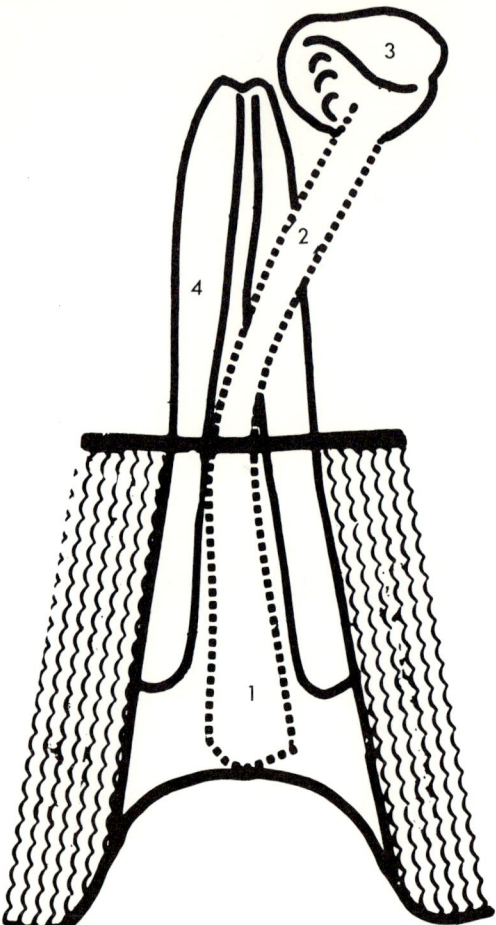

FIG. 12-1. Anatomy of penis. 1, Bulb of penis. 2, Corpus spongiosum. 3, Glans penis. 4, Corpus cavernosum.

nodes (mobile) are treated by dissection, sometimes after prior irradiation. Fixed nodes are usually treated with radiotherapy. Since nodal metastases indicate a poor prognosis, aggressive management is warranted.

The *technique of radiotherapy* for the treatment of the primary is seen in Fig. 12-2, where the penis is hung in a wax mold. Because of the small volume irradiated, conventional as well as more penetrating beams could be used. However, a gamma beam is preferable if the corpora are involved. The dose aimed at is about 6000 rads in about 6 weeks. Radium molds have been used successfully in the treatment of small lesions and they deliver 6000 to 7000 rads in 6 to 7 days. Skin reaction and perhaps a certain degree of radiation urethritis may occur, especially toward the end of treatment, but conservative measures and refrain from any instrumentation of the urethra may be all that is needed to allow the reaction to settle down.

The *prognosis* depends on the stage of the disease; a patient with a lesion limited to the skin has a 95% chance of cure. This figure drops to about 60% if the corpora are involved. Patients with mobile inguinal nodes stand a chance of 35% at a 5-year cure rate. The prognosis in patients with fixed nodes is very poor.

TESTIS

Malignant testicular tumors originate in the germ cell and are summarized in Table 12-1. However, our present discussion is limited to seminoma and embryonal carcinoma. It is worthwhile remembering that histological sections very often show a mixed pattern of the different types and "pure" tumors are rare. Tumors are usually classified and invariably behave according to the predominant tissue.

Testicular tumors have often been linked to trauma as a *predisposing factor*. They are more common in an undescended testis, and it is claimed that the change in the environmental temperature (that is, being higher in the abdomen) plays an important role in the *etiology*.

SEMINOMA

Seminoma forms about 60% of testicular malignancies and is more common in the fourth decade of life.

The tumor *spreads* mainly by lymphatics leading to early lymph node metastases. The ipsilateral iliac nodes are the first to be involved followed by the paraortic nodes. The contralateral pelvic nodes may be involved later on by way of crossing lymphatics. Locally, the tumor continues to be limited by the tunica albuginea testis (in-

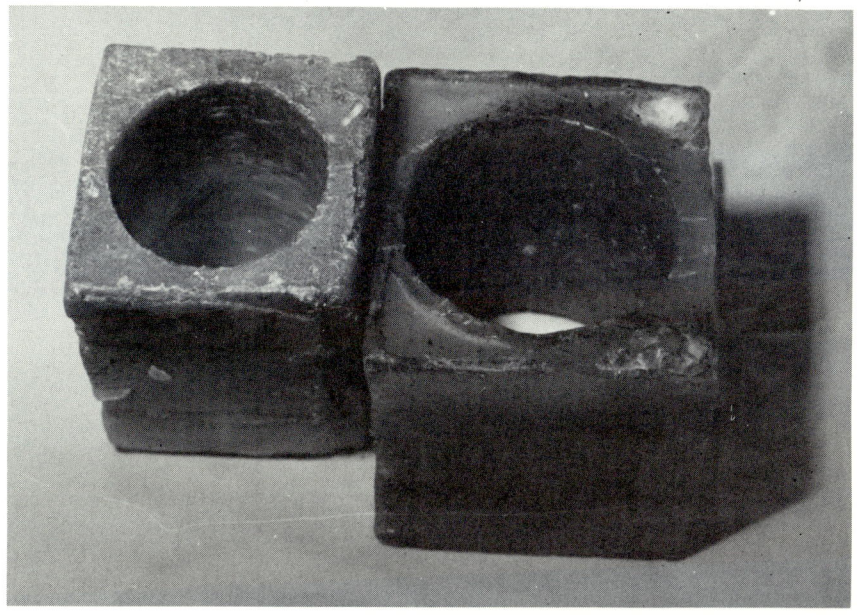

Fig. 12-2. Mold to treat penis.

TABLE 12-1. Malignant testicular tumors

Germ cells (97%)	Seminoma
	Embryonal carcinoma
	Malignant teratoma
	Choriocarcinoma
Nongerminal origin	Interstitial cell tumors
	Gonadostromal tumors

ner integument immediately covering the testis). Only rarely does the disease extend to involve the tunica vaginalis and beyond. Involvement of the tunica vaginalis or scrotum may herald inguinal node metastases. Bloodborne metastases to the lungs, bones, and splanchnic organs occur relatively late in the disease.

The usual *clinical picture* is that of heaviness of the testis or a testicular mass. Pain and gynecomastia may be the presenting symptom on rare occasions and are usually of bad prognostic significance. Rarely there is a hydrocele or a hematocele. A tumor in an undescended testis usually presents as an abdominal mass and may lead to the symptoms of an acute abdomen.

Exploration of any testicular swelling is the rule and is usually followed by orchiectomy. Other *investigations* of particular importance are lymphangiography and intravenous pyelography. Lymphangiography helps to identify the nodes (and their involvement) and thus to localize the treatment efforts. It also serves as a good indicator during the early follow-up period (when the nodes are still opacified by the retained dye).

The *treatment* of choice is orchiectomy through an inguinoscrotal incision and high ligation of the spermatic cord, followed by radiation therapy to the draining lymph nodes (iliac and paraortic). Seminoma is a very radiosensitive lesion and a dose of 3500 rads in 3½ weeks is enough to sterilize the tumor. During treatment the other testis as well as both kidneys should be protected adequately. If the paraortic nodes are involved, the mediastinal and supraclavicular nodes are also treated.

Chemotherapy by alkalating agents is employed when the disease is widely spread, though radiotherapy can often be

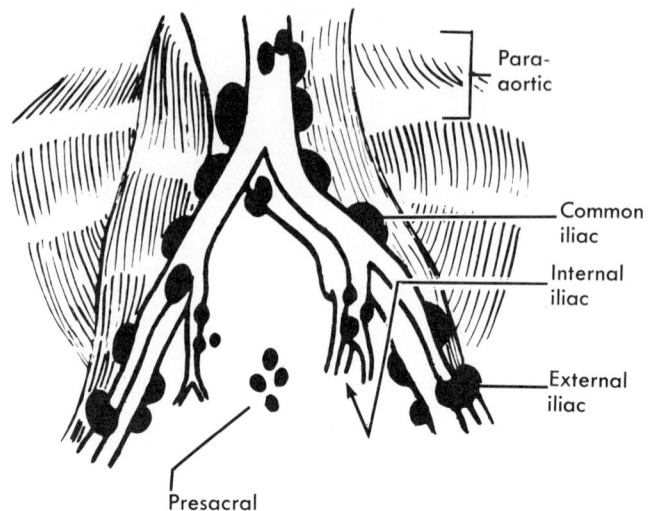
FIG. 12-3. Anatomy of iliac and para-aortic nodes.

used effectively to control various deposits because of the high radiosensitivity of the lesion.

The *technique* of radiotherapy is simple by use of a deeply penetrating beam (supervoltage x-ray beam) and large fields to irradiate the pelvic as well as the paraortic nodes (Fig. 12-3). The mediastinal nodes are treated only when the upper paraortic nodes are involved.

Complications of treatment like kidney damage or damage to the other testis should not be allowed to occur. However, some depression of the bone marrow may occur toward the end of the treatment, but the marrow usually recovers spontaneously after a few days' rest from treatment. Diarrhea may occur rarely and is easily controlled by simple measures.

Prognosis of seminoma is good, with a 3-year survival rate of about 90%. However, certain features worsen the prognosis; they are a lesion in an undescended testis, the presence of pain, gynecomastia, extensive nodal metastases, and a locally extensive lesion.

EMBRYONAL CARCINOMAS

The following represents the main points of difference between embryonal carcinoma and seminoma:

1. It is more common in younger patients (third decade of life).
2. The disease is less sensitive to radiotherapy than is seminoma, and a dose of 4500 rads in 4½ weeks to the lymph nodes is necessary.
3. The treatment is usually orchiectomy to the primary followed either by retroperitoneal node dissection or radiotherapy to the lymph nodes (up to a dose of 4500 rads) or combination of the two.
4. Prognosis is less favorable than in seminoma. The 5-year survival rate after orchiectomy and radiotherapy is about 60%. Results of orchiectomy and retroperitoneal node dissection is about 50%.

PROSTATE GLAND

Prostatic carcinoma represent the second most common site of malignancies in the male (lung, prostate, colon). It is predominantly a disease of the elderly and increases in incidence after the age of 50. There are no known predisposing factors, nor is there any connection between prostatic carcinoma and the benign hyperplasia of the prostate.

From its site of origin, the disease *spreads* to affect the rest of the prostate, and eventually it invades the capsule and extends to the surrounding structures. Bloodborne metastases to bones occur relatively early, and sometimes they form the presenting picture while the primary is quite small or even occult. Lymph node metastases to pelvic and paraortic nodes are known to occur with increasing frequency as the disease increases in stage.

Clinical staging of the disease is summarized as follows:

Stage A   Occult cancer
Stage B   Disease limited to the prostate with the capsule intact
Stage C   Involvement of the capsule and extension to surrounding tissues or confined within the capsule with elevation of serum acid phosphatase
Stage D   Disease with bone metastases or extrapelvic involvement

The main *pathological complication* is obstruction of the bladder neck followed by hydronephrosis and uremia in due course. However this complication occurs mostly in neglected cases. Repeated bleeding and resulting anemia may occur. Involvement of the rectum may lead to tenesmus and pain, which may also be caused by involvement of the presacral nerves.

In addition to the routine *investigations* intravenous pyelography and blood chemistry test are very important. Biopsy is usually obtained by a transurethral resection (TUR) or a needle biopsy (through the perineum or rectum). Open biopsy may be required in selected cases. A bone survey is important and sometimes a bone scan may be necessary. Lymphangiograms are made with increasing frequency now.

Until recently, *treatment* (of other than early stages) was mainly hormonal (by estrogens or orchiectomy, or both), but the results were so poor (20% 5-year survival rate) and cardiovascular complications were so high that other methods had to be evolved. These depend on the stage of the disease and the general condition of the patient (especially since most of them are elderly).

Stage A and B   If the patient is a good surgical risk, radical prostatectomy is recommended, but only 5% to 15% are eligible. If the patient is a poor risk or refuses the operation, external irradiation is used after a TUR if there is evidence of urinary obstruction.
Stage C   External irradiation follows a TUR if there is evidence of urinary obstruction.
Stage D   Employ palliative treatment by hormones if there is generalized pain in addition to radiation therapy to regions of metastases.

This policy is not fully accepted by all urologists yet, but the *results* achieved so far are extremely encouraging, with the 5-year survival rate free of disease being about 60%.

Technique of radiotherapy in the radical treatment of a prostatic carcinoma is rather important. A deeply penetrating "sharp" beam is mandatory (supervoltage x-ray beam). The fields are usually kept to a small size (8×8 to 10×10 cm.^{2}). Rotation (Fig. 3-16) or a multiple-fields plan is preferred in order to deliver the maximum dose to the prostate, with the dose to the rectum being kept minimal. The tumor dose aimed at is 6500 rads in 6½ weeks. Iliac nodes may be treated up to 4500 rads (in 4½ weeks) to sterilize subclinical disease.

Side effects of treatment are mainly rectal reaction (leading to diarrhea, tenesmus, and sometimes bleeding) and bladder-base reaction (dysuria, increased frequency of urination). Complications like radiation osteitis (and rarely fractures) of the pelvic bones should not be allowed to happen and are guarded against by careful planning. Rectal and bladder reactions usually respond to the same conservative measures described in the case of carcinoma of the cervix.

CHAPTER 13

URINARY SYSTEM

The urinary system is formed of two parts that differ greatly from each other: the kidney, whose functions are excretion and the reabsorption of the various components of urine, and the collecting and passage system (calyces and pelvis, ureters, bladder, and urethra). Tumors of the first are largely adenocarcinomas, whereas those of the latter are transitional cell carcinomas (arising from the lining transitional mucous membrane). The behavior and prognosis of both these types of tumors are completely different and are discussed separately.

KIDNEY

Table 13-1 shows a list of the different histological types of malignant tumors affecting the kidney. Our discussion is limited to renal cell carcinoma and nephroblastoma (Wilms' tumor), the two most common malignant kidney tumors. Nephroblastoma is discussed in Chapter 18, concerning childhood malignancies.

Renal cell carcinoma (hypernephroma)

Renal cell carcinomas form about 80% of malignant tumors of the kidney. They occur most commonly in men (2:1) in the fifth and sixth decades of life. There are two common histological types—the clear cell and the granular cell. Renal cell carcinoma *spreads* mainly by local invasion and by the hematogenous route. Locally the lesion extends from the renal cortex to the medulla and eventually involve the calyces. By outward growth it can involve the kidney capsule, the pericapsular fat, Gerota's capsule, and even the posterior abdominal muscles. Interestingly renal carcinomas extend along venous structures so that they not only spread (often and early) by the hematological route (to lungs and bones) but also may grow along the renal vein into the inferior vena cava as a finger inside a glove. Lymph node metastases were believed to be infrequent, but recent publications claim that they occur in about 25% of the cases distributed at the renal pedicle, along the renal vein and paraortic region.

Renal cell carcinoma is characterized by displaying a varied and somewhat unexpected *clinical picture*. The patient may suffer from general symptoms like fever, anemia (even without hematuria), weakness, and loss of weight. However, hematuria is the commonest presenting picture (70%) followed by flank pain (50%) and a palpable mass. On the other hand, the incidental discovery of a pulmonary nodule or abnormality in a routine intravenous pyelogram may be the only signs manifested.

Besides routine laboratory *investigations*,

TABLE 13-1. Primary kidney tumors

Benign	Malignant
Fibroma (capsule)	Fibrosarcoma
Adenoma	Adenocarcinoma (hypernephroma)
	Adenomyosarcoma or embryonal kidney tumors or Wilms' tumor
Hamartoma	
Leiomyoma	Leiomyosarcoma
Lipoma	Liposarcoma
Papilloma (urothelium*)	Transitional carcinoma (urothelium)
	Squamous cell carcinoma (urothelium)

*Urothelium includes renal pelvis, ureters, bladder, and urethra.

an intravenous pyelogram, a nephrotomogram, and a selective renal angiogram are of prime importance in confirming the diagnosis, and an inferior vena cavagram (to detect spread along the inferior vena cava) and a lymphangiogram can be of help in assessing the spread of the disease. A routine urine cytological test may provide sufficient evidence of positive diagnosis in certain cases.

The *treatment of the primary* is usually nephrectomy (preferably radical nephrectomy through a transabdominal route). The place of radiotherapy in treating the primary is still controversial and it may be summarized as follows:

Preoperative radiotherapy is claimed by some authors (Riches, Windeyer) to improve the results of treatment by sterilizing the most malignant cells and thus diminishing the chances of widespread metastases and local recurrence. It may also lead to reduction in the size of the lesion and therefore convert an otherwise unresectable tumor. A major objection to preoperative radiotherapy is that histological proof of malignancy is unavailable prior to treatment. However present-day angiography and nephrotomography have a high enough diagnostic accuracy so as to preclude the need for histological confirmation.

The *technique* of radiotherapy usually involves two opposing fields. A deeply penetrating beam (gamma or supervoltage x-ray beam) is important. The dose aimed at is usually 4000 to 4500 rads in 4 to 5 weeks. Because the treatment volume is large, some patients may suffer from radiation sickness, especially when the right kidney is treated (since the liver is included in the treatment volume). Diarrhea and colonic cramps may be troublesome, but these are corrected with simple measures.

Postoperative radiotherapy. This is especially recommended if the capsule or surrounding tissues are involved. Lymphatic involvement and extension to the renal pelvis are two other indications. The technique may be seen in Fig. 13-1, where the renal bed as well as the lymph nodes are included. Such a plan delivers minimal irradiation to neighboring vital structures, the spinal cord and the contralateral kidney (structures very sensitive to radiation). The dose aimed at is 5000 rads in 5 weeks.

Prognosis depends on the extension of the disease, with earlier lesions displaying a more favorable picture than do later ones (which show invasion of renal capsule or vein); their respective 5-year survival rates are 40% and 10%. Radical nephrectomy (with dissection of regional lymph nodes) has more favorable results than does simple nephrectomy (60% and 40%, respectively).

BLADDER AND UROTHELIUM

Lesions that affect the renal pelvis, ureters, bladder, and urethra are histologically

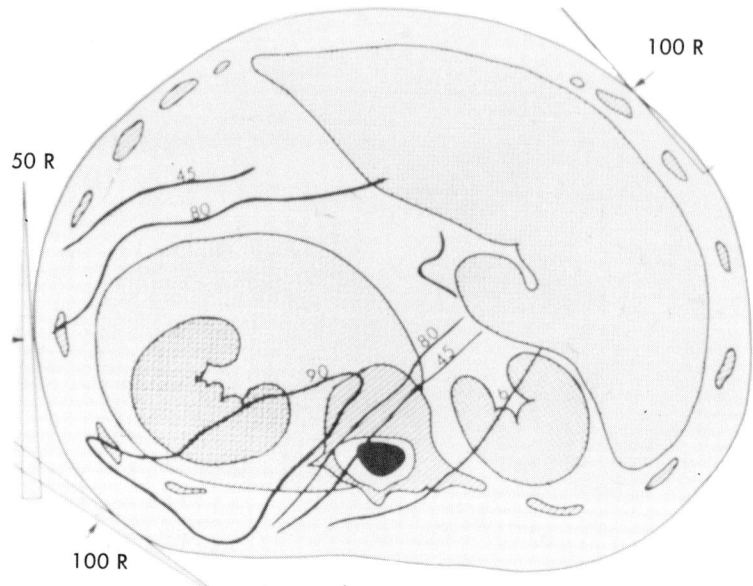

Fig. 13-1. Technique of postoperative treatment after nephrectomy for renal cell carcinoma.

the same and behave similarly except for the effect of the tumor bed. The following list shows the different histological types of primary bladder malignancies:

Epithelium
  Transitional cell carcinoma
  Squamous cell carcinoma
  Adenocarcinoma from the following:
    Paraurethral glands
    Paraprostatic glands
    Cystitis glandularis
    Adenofibroma
    Urachal or cloacal glands
    Endometriosis
Muscle
  Myosarcoma (leiomyosarcoma and rhabdomyosarcoma)
Rare tumors
  Myxosarcoma
  Osteochondrosarcoma
  Lymphosarcoma

Our discussion is limited to transitional cell carcinoma, which represents over 90% of the total. Bladder carcinoma is the most frequent malignant tumor of the urinary tract and occurs in men (2.3:1) in their fifth and sixth decades of life.

These lesions are strongly linked to carcinogens in certain aromatic amines like aniline dyes, which were used extensively in the printing industry. The tumor is more common in workers in rubber and cable industries. Chronic irritation, such as occurs with bilharziasis *(Schistosoma haematobium)* and stones, is another *predisposing factor*. Furthermore, tumors that follow chronic irritation are predominantly squamous cell carcinomas (especially in the renal pelvis). Leukoplakia, congenital extrophy and vesical diverticula are other less known etiological factors.

Bladder lesions usually originate in the mucous membrane of the bladder trigone and lateral walls. It *spreads* mainly by local invasion to the muscle layer, paravesical tissues, and prostate gland. The lesion may extend to the pelvic walls in its late stages. Lymph node metastases increase as the disease invades the muscular layers (and their lymphatics) or beyond. The nodes involved are the iliac followed by the paraortic ones. Bloodborne metastases are rare, but they are being seen more frequently nowadays, since local treatment is more successful and patients live longer.

Clinical staging of bladder carcinomas depend on the extent of the disease as assessed clinically by cystoscopy and bimanual examinations under general anesthesia (to afford complete relaxation) in addition to an intravenous pyelogram. Since there is no internationally accepted staging the following is the most widely used:

Stage 0	Disease limited to superficial mucosa
Stage A	Disease with submucosal infiltration
Stage B1	Disease involving the superficial muscle layer
Stage B2	Disease involving the deep muscle layer
Stage C	Disease with perivesical infiltration
Stage D	Disease fixed to pelvic wall or involving the prostate

The histological grade of the lesion usually indicates its malignancy and thus its potential of spread. Lesions graded as III or IV are usually much more widely spread than are those graded as I or II.

The most common presenting *clinical picture* is hematuria associated with frequency and dysurea. Back pain may be present especially in advanced obstructive (of ureter and urethra) lesions or where the presacral nerves are involved.

Cystoscopy, examination under anesthesia (rectal examination), biopsy, and intravenous pyelography are the most important *investigations*. The last indicates the anatomical and functional condition of the ureters and the kidneys. Blood chemistry especially urea and creatinine levels are important.

Treatment depends on the stage of the lesion, its size, and its site in the bladder. The most salient features are summarized as follows:

Stage A	*Small lesions* (even if multiple) are treated by transurethral cauterization provided that the biopsy shows a well-differentiated picture.
Stage A	*Diffuse lesions* (not amenable to cautery) are treated either by total cystectomy or external irradiation aimed at the whole bladder. If the lesions are anaplastic the whole pelvis is irradiated.
Stage B1	*Small lesion* (1) Partial cystectomy especially if it is in the bladder dome; a margin of ½ inch should be excised (2) Cystotomy, cautery, and interstitial implant if partial cystectomy not possible (3) External irradiation to bladder can correct the disease *Large lesion* or multiple lesions; total cystectomy or external irradiation to the whole pelvis.
Stage B2 and C	Preoperative external irradiation (4000 rads) is followed by total cystectomy. Some authors recommend surgery or radiotherapy alone but the results of either alone are poor.
Stage D	Palliative treatment involves radiotherapy for bleeding and pain, and surgery by transurethral resection for obstruction.

Technique of radiotherapy

If an *interstitial implant* is to be permanent, use gold grains; but if it is to be temporary, use tantalum wires. The two techniques are described on p. 21. The dose aimed at should be about 6500 rads.

If *external irradiation* is to be employed, two techniques are generally involved. The first is aimed at treating the bladder and paravesical tissues only (Fig. 13-2). The dose aimed at is usually about 6000 to 6500 rads in 6 to 7 weeks. Supervoltage x-ray or a gamma beam of high penetration is necessary. The second technique is that aimed at treating the whole pelvis including the regional nodes (Fig. 13-3), where the fields and the integral doses are larger.

Complications of radiotherapy

Patients receiving radical radiotherapy (6000 rads) may suffer from cystitis with aggravation of some of their symptoms, especially dysurea and frequency. Diarrhea and bowel reaction may also occur on occasions. It may be wise to keep these patients on urinary antibiotics and antispasmodics, especially during the latter part of treatment. This is specifically indicated in patients with irritable or infected bladder

132 *Clinical radiation oncology*

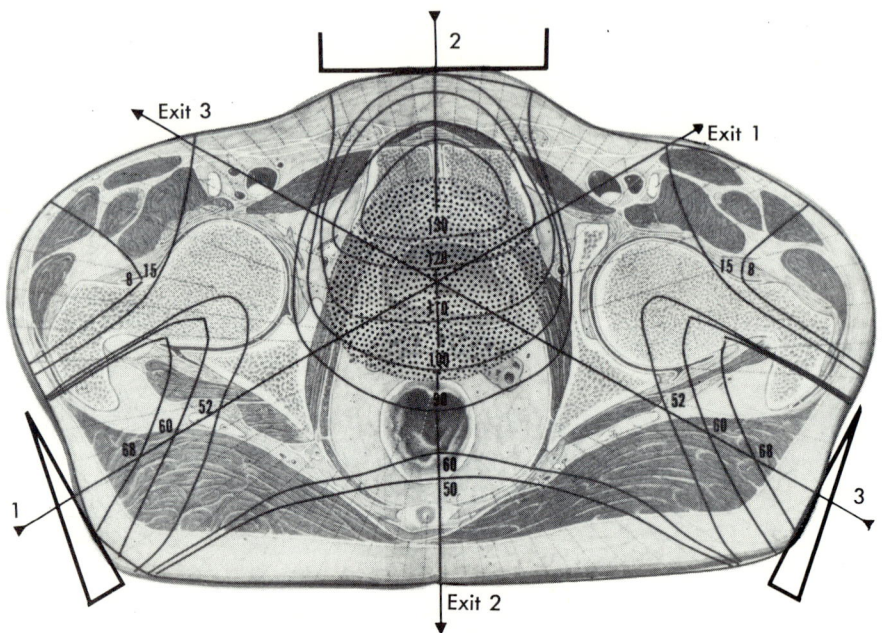

Fig. 13-2. Technique of treating around the bladder and paravesically.

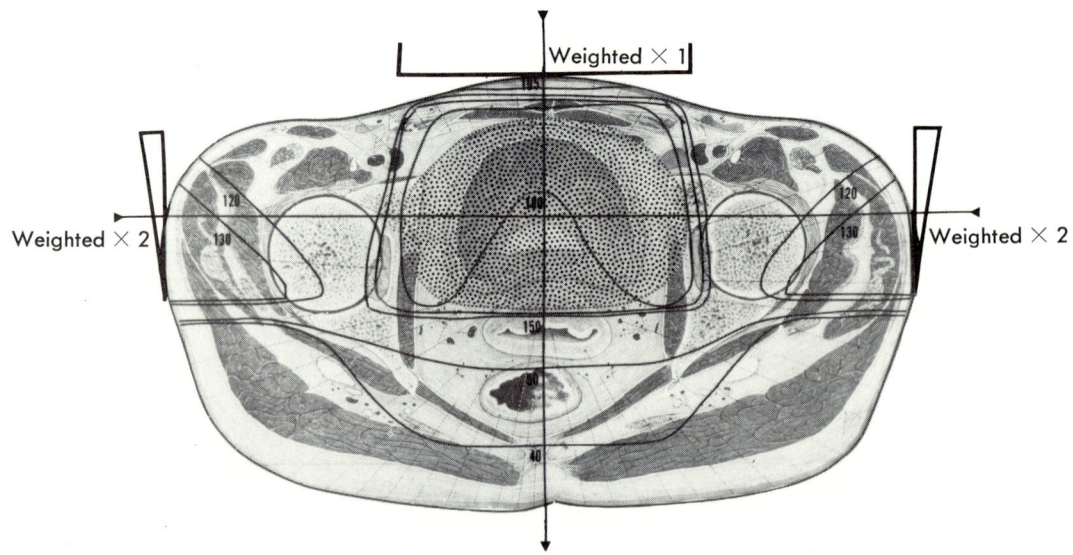

Fig. 13-3. Technique of treating the whole pelvis around the bladder.

or those who underwent recent multiple cauteries before being referred to radiotherapy.

In some publications prognosis has been related to the method of treatment, whereas it is probably more related to the stage of the disease at presentation provided that the disease is treated adequately.

In stage A the 5-year survival rate is about 80%, especially when the lesions are small and limited in number. The figure drops to about 65% in stage B1. The best results achieved in stages B2 and C so far are those of combined approach (preoperative radiotherapy followed by surgery) and amount to a 36% 5-year survival rate. The results of surgery alone are about 20%.

CHAPTER 14

LYMPHORETICULAR SYSTEM

Lymphoreticular tissue is widely spread all over the body and is found in different organs with varying degrees of abundance. However lymph nodes and areas rich in accumulations of lymphoid tissue (such as tonsils or posterior third of the tongue) represent stations for lymph drainage as well as for carrying other functions of the system (such as immunoreactivity). It follows that malignant tumors originating in lymphoreticular tissues can occur in any region or organ, but they are most common in lymph nodes and areas of lymphoid tissue accumulations. Figs. 14-1 and 9-2 show the anatomy of the most prominent nodes, and it helps the reader to formulate an idea about the extent of this system. Discussion is concentrated on the three most common —Hodgkin's lymphoma and of the non-Hodgkin lymphomas: lymphosarcoma and reticulum cell sarcoma.

HODGKIN'S DISEASE

This disease, named after Thomas Hodgkin, consists of many histological types, which vary in behavior as well as prognosis. An existing controversy around the pathological classification has been settled for the most part and the one used below represents the histological types and their incidence:
Hodgkin's disease
Lymphocyte predominance 5%
Nodular sclerosis 52%
Mixed cellularity 37%
Lymphocyte depletion 6%

The limitation of this text does not allow detailed discussion of the many pertinent findings regarding the significance of the histological classification; suffice it to say that the types shown above are arranged in order of increasing degrees of malignancy (the 5-year survival rate is 90%, 70%, 33%, and 10%, respectively). Not only is prognosis indicated by this classification, but it also allows selection of proper clinical management.

Hodgkin's lymphoma forms about 40% of all malignant lymphomas. It is more common in the third decade of life especially the lymphocyte-predominant variety. The lymphocyte-depleted variety is more common in older age groups (fifth and sixth decades). The disease is more common in males (4:3).

For many decades controversy raged around the multiplicity of lymph node involvement, which characterizes this dis-

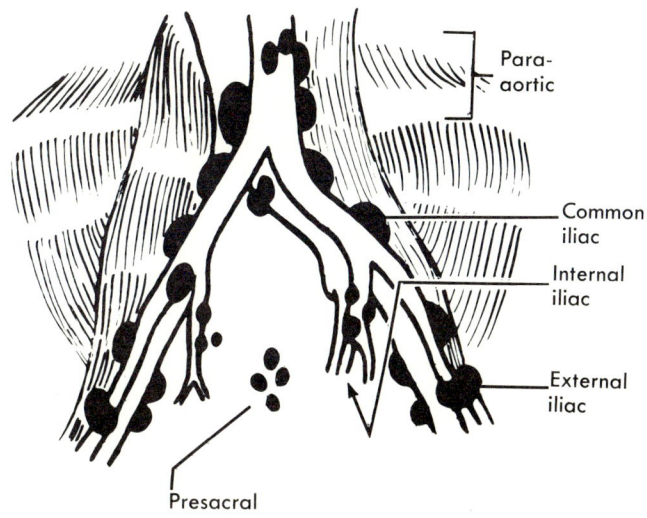

FIG. 14-1. Para-aortic and iliac nodal stations.

ease, and whether it is a sign of systematic *spread* from one region to the other or an evidence of multifocal origin. Be that as it may, the most common method of progress of the disease is by lymph node involvement, whether systematic (that is, one group to an adjoining one) or distant. The disease continues to be limited to lymph nodes for a relatively long time, but eventually it spreads to other organs, especially the spleen, liver, bone marrow, and lungs.

Clinical staging has evolved as a very important factor in assessing the prognosis of the disease and thus serving as a valid parameter for treatment protocols. Staging depends on clinical findings as well as certain *investigations* such as chest x-ray films and tomograms, lymphangiography, bone marrow biopsy, and more recently laparotomy (including splenectomy and lymph node biopsy). Lymph node biopsy is often essential to establish the diagnosis. Skin tests for delayed hypersensitivity (cutaneous anergy is common in the lymphocyte-depletion type) demonstrates the state of altered immunity and may serve as an indicator to progress of disease or response to treatment. The following staging system is not internationally adopted, though widely accepted:

Stage I   Disease limited to one lymph node group
Stage II   Disease limited to two (or more) lymph node groups on one side of the diaphragm
Stage III Disease affecting nodes on both sides of the diaphragm
Stage IV   Disease affecting organs other than nodes by metastatic spread (such as liver, lungs, bones, multiple skin nodules)

Each of these stages is classified into A or B depending on whether or not the patient is suffering from generalized symptoms (fever, weight loss, night sweats).

The classical *clinical picture* of Hodgkin's lymphoma is a young patient presenting usually with enlarged cervical nodes (in about 70% of cases). This may be accompanied with fever, night sweats, pruritus, or loss of weight. Less often the patient presents with *pathological complications,* such as anemia (from bone marrow replacement), superior mediastinal obstruction (from the pressure of a mediastinal mass on the superior vena cava and surrounding structures), or edema of a limb (from massive lymph node involvement). An equally rare presenting clinical picture is that of primary organ involvement by Hodgkin's lymphoma (designated by *e* in clinical staging), such as dyspeptic symptoms caused by primary stomach Hodgkin's disease, proptosis caused by orbital disease, or nasal obstruction caused by nasopharyngeal involvement. Occasionally an isolated tumor deposit may exist in an organ adjacent to nodal disease, such a pulmonary deposit with hilar nodes.

Hodgkin's lymphoma is a highly radiosensitive disease and therefore radiotherapy is the *treatment* of choice. The disease is also amenable to chemotherapeutic agents, which may be used in various combination with radiotherapy.

The treatment of Hodgkin's disease depends primarily on the clinical stage of the disease, with recognition of the fact that more malignant histological types are likely to be widely spread than the relatively more favorable ones. Although there is general agreement that the primary treatment for stages I and II is radiation therapy, no such accord exists regarding the volume of nodes to be irradiated. Some authors recommend total nodal irradiation in stages I and II, whereas others recommend an upper mantle-shaped field or a lower inverted-Y field for stage I in above or below the diaphragm respectively. Moreover, splenectomy is considered by some as a necessary investigation and first step of treatment in all cases. Since involvement of the spleen would put the case in stage III (with a different prognosis and treatment), those authors claim that laparotomy and splenectomy make up the only sure method to achieve this. Stage III is treated by total nodal irradiation in addition to cytotoxic agents, especially when there are systemic symptoms (stage III B). Stage IV is treated primarily by various combinations of the available cytotoxic agents (nitrogen mustard, cyclophosphamide [Cytoxan], vinblastine, procarbazine, corticosteroids, 1,3-bis(2-chloroethyl)-1-nitrosourea [BCNU]), in addition to radiation therapy

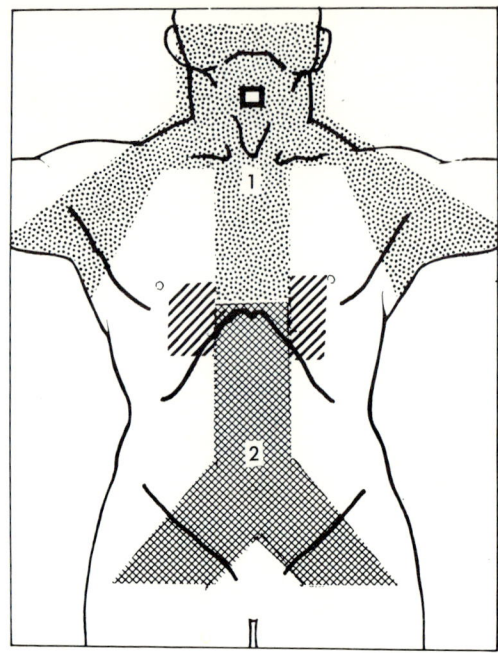

Fig. 14-2. Field to treat mantle and Y-shaped field. (A splenic portal may be added.)

aimed at relieving specific symptoms, such as treatment of the mediastinum to relieve superior mediastinal obstruction.

The technique of radiotherapy calls for a deeply penetrating beam (supervoltage x-ray beam or gamma beam) and a treatment distance (source-to-skin distance) capable of producing a large field to cover an upper mantle-shaped field or a lower inverted-Y field (Fig. 14-2). The dose aimed at is about 4000 rads in 4 weeks.

The most important side affect of treatment is the depression of bone marrow, especially the white cells (leading to leukopenia). This is especially noticeable in total nodal irradiation. It is more severe when the spleen is included in the treatment volume. This is another reason used by the authors who recommend splenectomy to support their argument. General constitutional disturbances, such as nausea and loss of appetite, may be noticed especially in older patients.

Dysphagia from radiation esophagitis (during the treatment of the mediastinum) may be troublesome on rare occasions, but it can be relieved by the use of mucilages (aspirin mucilage or xylocaine 1%). Sensitive structures like the kidney and spinal cord must be protected against excessive irradiation.

The *prognosis* of this disease has undergone a revolution in the last few years from a relatively hopeless disease to a curable one. The 5-year survival figures are around 85% in stage I and 65% in stage II. Only about 35% to 40% of those suffering from stage III disease live for 5 years, and about 20% of stage IV patients do the same. Stage for stage the patients with an A classification have a 15% to 30% higher survival compared to those with B classification. Recent aggressive multidrug chemotherapy has improved the results of stages IIIB and IV with about half the patients surviving for 5 years. Obviously there is still a great room for improvement in the results of treatment, especially in the advanced stages.

NON-HODGKIN LYMPHOMAS

Lymphosarcoma and reticulum cell sarcoma are the two main types in this category. This nomenclature has been superseded by the histological classification, a simplified version of which is shown below.

	Nodular	*Diffuse*
Lympho-sarcoma	Nodular lymphocytic, well differentiated	Diffuse lymphocytic, well differentiated
	Nodular lymphocytic, poorly differentiated	Diffuse lymphocytic, poorly differentiated
		Diffuse undifferentiated
Reticulum cell sarcoma	Nodular mixed histiocytic lymphocytic	Diffuse mixed histiocytic lymphocytic
	Nodular histiocytic	Diffuse histiocytic

As a result of experience gained from the treatment of Hodgkin's disease, the need for clinical staging became apparent. However, because there are many similarities between both Hodgkin's and non-Hodgkin lymphomas, a parallel clinical staging system has been adopted. Nevertheless there are still several salient features of non-Hodgkin lymphomas. They are summarized as follows:

1. Lymphosarcomas represent about 40% of malignant lymphomas. Reticulum cell sarcomas form about 20%.

2. The most common age is the fifth and sixth decades of life. Both are somewhat more common in men.

3. Of the several types of lymphosarcomas, the nodular well-differentiated lymphocytic variety has the best prognosis. Diffuse lymphocytic poorly differentiated lymphomas possess more malignant features and have a much less favorable prognosis. In advanced stages of lymphosarcomas some patients may develop lymphatic leukemia. On the other hand, reticulum cell sarcomas or the histiocytic lymphomas are more malignant than the group of lymphosarcomas.

4. The origin and spread of lymphosarcomas and reticulum cell sarcomas is generally similar to Hodgkin's although these non-Hodgkin types have a more widespread disease pattern. A relatively high percentage of reticulum cell sarcomas have an extranodal origin, with retroperitoneal tissues and bone being among the common sites.

5. Both lymphosarcomas and reticulum cell sarcomas are radiosensitive lesions, with the former being more so. The treatment of choice of the primary lesion is radiation therapy. The role of surgery is usually limited to exploration and biopsy. However on certain occasions, the excision of the organ carrying the lesion is recommended; for example, resection of a loop of intestine (carrying a lesion) may be the best line of management.

The *role of chemotherapy* is undisputed in disseminated cases of lymphosarcomas and reticulum cell sarcomas. However, recently cytotoxic drugs have been used in combination with radiotherapy for relatively early stages.

The *technique of radiotherapy* utilizes

large fields to include all the lymph nodes in one region. Recent trials of treatment techniques similar to those used in Hodgkin's disease are in progress. The dose recommended is 4000 to 4500 rads in 4½ weeks, with the higher dose utilized in cases of reticulum cell sarcoma. Total body irradiation is being tried in some centers for the treatment of diffuse disease. Side effects of treatment and their management are the same as in Hodgkin's disease.

Prognosis is more favorable in lymphosarcomas compared to reticulum cell sarcomas. The 5-year survival rate of patients suffering from the former is about 40%, whereas it is about 25% for the latter. Early cases of lymphosarcoma fare much better than do late ones (70% compared to 16%).

CHAPTER 15

CENTRAL NERVOUS SYSTEM

Tumors of the central nervous system are unique in that they are locally invasive and metastasize outside the cerebrospinal axis only on very rare occasions. Moreover, apart from medulloblastoma and ependymoma, they continue to be limited to their site of origin. Medulloblastoma and ependymoma may metastasize throughout the ventricular system (inside the brain) as well as seed the spinal canal. Nevertheless the majority of tumors of the central nervous system run a very malignant course by virtue of their proximity to vital structures. Moreover, as all these tumors grow in areas where the surrounding bony calvarium precludes expansion, tissues may be damaged just by displacement and herniation. Thus, the term "space-occupying lesion" evolved and expresses the mechanism behind the clinical picture.

Primary tumors of the central nervous system
    Tumors of congenital origin
        Chordoma
        Craniopharyngioma
        Colloid cysts of third ventricle
        Mixed tumors (cholesteatoma)
    Tumors of the meninges
        Meningioma
        Melanoma
    Tumors of the supporting connective tissue (glial)
        Astrocytomas (grades I to IV)
        Oligodendroglioma
        Ependymoma (related to ependymal cells of ventricles)
        Medulloblastoma
    Tumors of nerve cells
        Neurocytoma
        Neuroblastoma
        Retinoblastoma
    Tumors of extramedullary neurogenic tumors
        Supporting cells
            Schwannoma
            Acoustic neurinoma
            Multiple neurofibromatosis
            Neurogenic sarcoma
        Peripheral nerves
            Ganglioneuroma
            Plexiform neuroma
            Neuroblastoma and sympatheticoblastoma
            Neurofibroma
        Miscellaneous
            Pheochromocytoma
            Carotid body tumor
    Tumors of vascular and perivascular tissue
        Hemangioendothelioma
        Hemangiosarcoma
        Sarcoma
    Pineal tumors
    Hypophyseal tumors
        Chromophobe adenoma
        Acidophil adenoma
        Basophil adenoma
Metastatic tumors of the central nervous system

The preceding outline lists the tumors that affect the central nervous system, but our discussion is limited to gliomas, pituitary tumors, and metastatic lesions. Medulloblastomas and craniopharyngiomas are discussed under the heading "childhood tumors."

GLIOMAS (ASTROCYTOMAS)

Gliomas form about half of all the tumors of the central nervous system. They arise from the glial cells, or astrocytes (supporting or "connective" tissue of the brain). They occur with almost equal frequency in both sexes around the fourth, fifth, and sixth decades of life. However, gliomas of the brainstem and cerebellum are more common in children around 4 years of age.

The histological appearance of gliomas is characterized by great variability. They are *classified* into four grades of the following pattern: A grade I astrocytoma (or glioma) is a very well defined lesion, whereas a grade IV astrocytoma (glioblastoma multiforme) is very anaplastic, highly invasive, and very poorly defined. Astrocytomas graded II and III possess intermediate characteristics. Oligodendroglioma is a well-defined glioma (grade I astrocytoma) that arises from the oligodendroglial cells.

Gliomas *spread* almost exclusively by local expansion and invasion. Grades I and II astrocytomas spread mainly by expansion, whereas grades III and IV invade surrounding structures. However, they are usually contained by the pia mater (innermost meningeal covering).

The *pathological complications* and clinical picture of gliomas depend mainly on the site of origin of the tumor and its size. The tumor size underlies the incidence of the so-called general symptoms and signs, whereas the site dictates the specific clinical picture of a particular lesion. The general symptoms are attributable to increased intracranial tension and are summarized as follows: headache, vomiting, dizziness, and papilledema or choking of the optic disk (associated with engorged retinal veins and hemorrhages caused by obstruction of the optic vein). This picture is not related to the site of the tumor, but rather to its

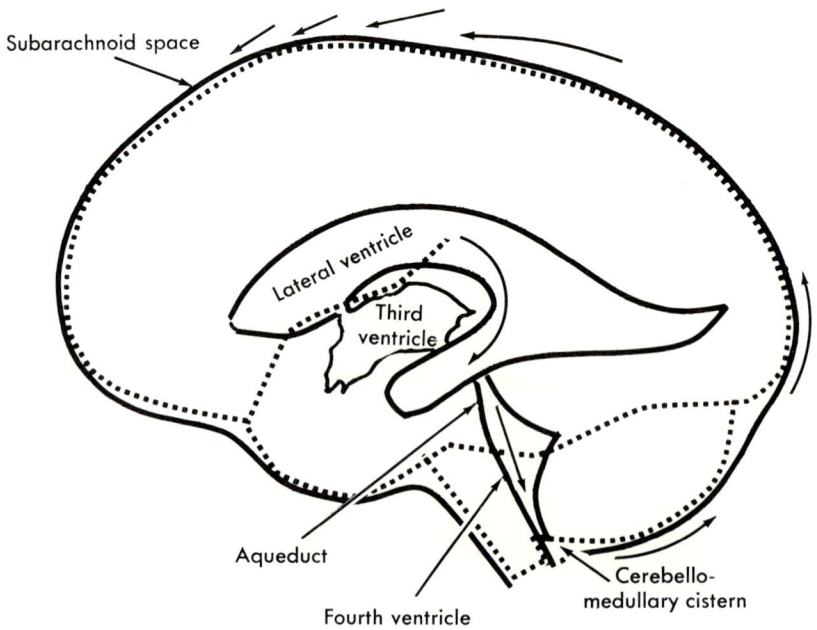

Fig. 15-1. Cerebrospinal fluid pathways.

effect on the intracranial pressure. Any obstruction to venous return or the circulation of cerebrospinal fluid (Fig. 15-1) can lead to increased intracranial pressure. Therefore, tumors obstructing the third ventricle, aqueduct, fourth ventricle, or the foramina are more likely (and earlier) to demonstrate this picture than those in the cerebrum, especially the frontal or frontoparietal regions.

LOCALIZING SYMPTOMS

Localizing symptoms depend mainly on the site of a particular lesion and the nerve fibers affected. However, epileptic fits may occur regardless of the specific site. On occasions, there may be a special prodrome (symptoms or signs preceding the epileptic fit), or a jacksonian type of attack (where the attack is localized to a certain organ or extremity, such as an arm), which may denote the site of the origin of the tumors.

It is impossible to mention all the localizing symptoms in a work of this scope, but a glance at Figs. 15-2 and 15-3 will give one some idea.

Tumors of the frontal lobe can be silent, that is, without any localizing symptoms for a long time. Changes in personality, behavior, and memory may be the only symptoms.

Tumors of the parietal lobe demonstrate a variable picture depending on the exact site. Deficiency of the motor functions (such as paresis or paralysis) of a limb or a group of muscles may be the main presenting picture if the tumor is limited to the precentral gyrus. If the lesion is situated somewhat posteriorly (postcentral gyrus), the main deficit may be sensory, especially the highly developed sensations (as opposed to pain and temperature, which are localized in the thalamic regions).

Tumors of the occipital lobe are usually characterized by visual disturbances as a result of interruption of the visual pathways and visual centers. Tumors of the *temporal lobe* may cause changes in the sense of smell and faculty of speech. A syndrome of temporal lobe epilepsy may be present in some cases. *Tumors of the posterior cranial fossa and cerebellum* usually lead to loss of balance, abnormal characteristic speech (staccato), and loss of muscular tone, in addition to early signs of increased intracranial tension (if the lesion is situated near the fourth ventricle).

Investigations of brain tumors are quite elaborate, and it is possible in most cases to almost pinpoint the lesion before the operation. In addition to a cerebrospinal fluid examination (to detect an increase in proteins or an abnormal cytological condition) and electroencephalography (to detect any change in brain waves that may be characteristic of tumors of certain sites), brain scans (using ^{99m}Tc-pertechnetate) and cerebral angiograms are done in this sequence. Brain scans are used as screening tests because of their safety, simplicity, and reliability.

Cerebral angiograms (usually carotid angiograms) may show the arterial as well as the venous circulation of the tumor, either or both of which may be pathognomonic of disease. Air studies (pneumoencephalograms) are helpful for delineation of tumors situated centrally in and about the ventricular system and parapituitary area. Ventricular and cisternal pneumoencephalograms are more hazardous, and on certain occasions they should be done in the immediate preoperative period.

Treatment of gliomas involves a primary exploration by craniotomy and complete removal if possible. Where blockage of the circulation of cerebrospinal fluid exists and where tumor removal is not possible, a shunt is established to produce drainage. The shunt may be between the ventricle above the obstruction and cisterns below it or between the ventricle and a large vein or the right cardiac atrium. However, surgical extirpation is not possible if the tumor is situated in the brainstem region (cerebral peduncles, pons, medulla) or corpus callosum because any disturb-

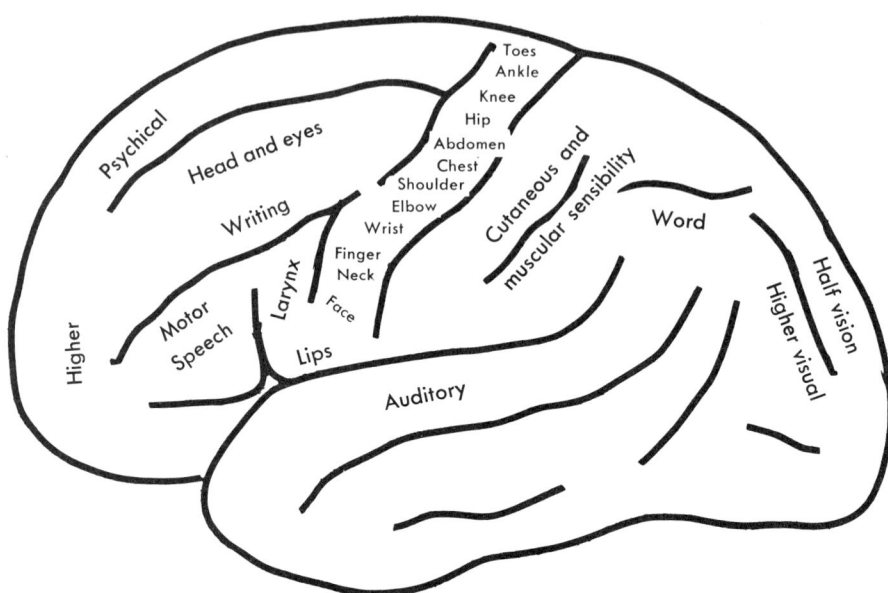

FIG. 15-2. Diagram of localization of function in different parts of the cortex.

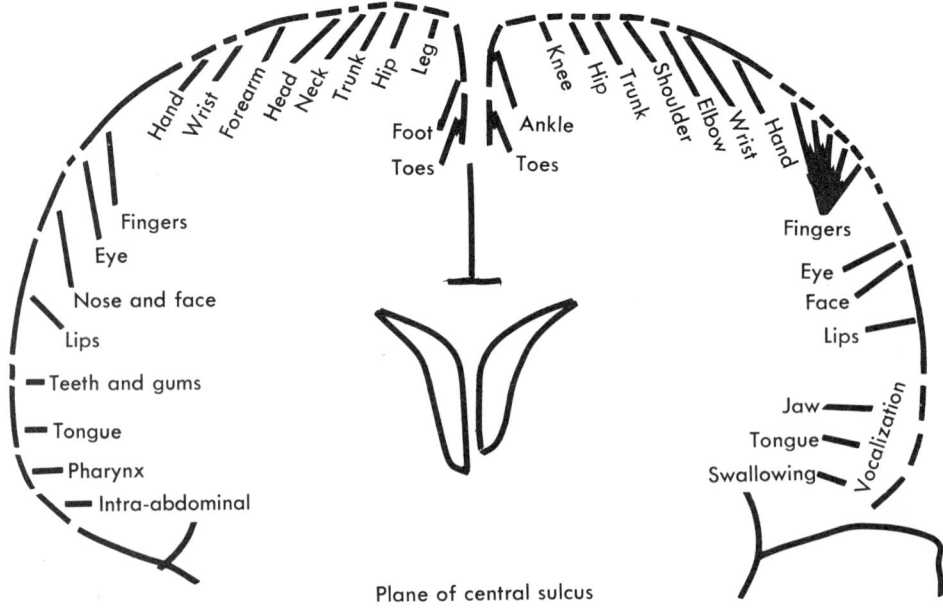

FIG. 15-3. Diagram of localization in motor *(left)* and sensory cortex *(right)*.

ance of these anatomical regions may prove extremely damaging or even fatal. Radiotherapy may be given in these occasions without tissue diagnosis. In cases where craniotomy and removal of the tumor has been done, postoperative radiotherapy is recommended for grades III and IV astrocytomas.

The *technique of radiotherapy* calls for a deeply penetrating beam. Field arrangements depend on the size and site of the lesion. It may be advisable to start with a larger field to deliver a dose of 4000 to 4500 rads in about 5 weeks, after which fields are reduced in size to concentrate the treatment on the immediate tumor volume (which should be either marked by silver clips at the time of operation or delineated from previous angiography) for a further 1000 rads in about 1 week.

Side effects of such a course of management are usually limited to temporary epilation of scalp hair, but mild general effects may occasionally occur. On rare occasions, a certain degree of brain edema (and worsening of signs and symptoms of increased intracranial tension) may occur, especially if large doses are given at the beginning of treatment in the presence of residual increased intracranial tension. Lack of a shunt or obstruction of the shunting catheter to relieve such tension may predispose to such an incident. Prednisone and diuretics may relieve this condition, but reoperation and establishing an effective shunt may be necessary on rare occasions.

Prognosis of astrocytomas either as to survival of the patient or as to a satisfactory functional result depends on the grade as well as the site of the lesion (those of silent brain regions are most favorable) and the degree of neurological damage at presentation (mild paresis as compared to distinct paralysis). Provided that the site of the lesion and the degree of neurological damage at presentation are not critical, grade I astrocytomas are curable. On the other hand, the 5-year survival figures of grade IV astrocytomas (glioblastoma multiforme) are very poor, 5% to 10%. The 5-year survival rate of grade II is about 35%.

METASTATIC BRAIN LESIONS

Metastatic brain lesions form about 10% to 20% of all intracranial neoplasms. Bronchogenic carcinoma is the most common primary lesion (about 60%) followed by that of the breast, pancreas, lower intestine, and kidney and finally malignant melanoma, but no malignancy is exempt. They are most common around the sixth decade of life, except when they originate from tumors of the young (such as testicular tumors).

Histology of the brain metastases would depend on the lesion of origin and very often reproduces it so that the primary site is identifiable. The *clinical picture* as well as pathological complications are very similar to those of gliomas. In fact it is impossible in some cases to differentiate between metastatic lesions and primary gliomas except on the basis of the history of previous malignancy. *Investigations* including brain scans and angiograms may reveal more than one lesion; such a condition is almost pathognomonic of metastases. However, in cases where solitary brain metastases make the presenting picture without a previously diagnosed primary lesion (such as in some renal cell or bronchial carcinomas), biopsy is the only method of diagnosis.

Treatment is usually a combination of steroids and radiation therapy to the whole brain. Occasionally excision of a single metastatic lesion (such as in renal cell carcinoma) may be enough but the usual multiplicity of the lesions limits the success of such an approach.

The *technique of radiotherapy* is quite simple; it uses two large opposing fields to treat the whole brain, including the cerebellum. The optimal dose is unresolved but it ranges from 3000 rads in 2 weeks to 4500 in 5 weeks. This is usually carried out without any undesirable side effects.

Prognosis

It is estimated that about three fourths of the patients treated benefit from the treatment with disappearance of their symptoms and correction of the neurological deficits. However, the latter may be only partial, and patients are left with some residual disability depending on the site of the metastasis and the degree of damage at presentation. The length of response varies, but only a fraction of the patients who respond live for over 1 year. On rare occasions, recurrence of symptoms may be associated with evidence of regrowth of the brain lesion (as demonstrated by brain scan), and it may be possible to retreat the patient with a short course of radiotherapy (delivering a smaller dose), but response is usually limited.

PITUITARY TUMORS

Pituitary adenomas form about 15% of all intracranial tumors and arise from the anterior lobe of the gland. There are three types—chromophobe, eosinophil (chromophil), and basophil. Chromophobe adenomas are the most common tumors, occur commonly in adulthood, and are of equal incidence in both sexes.

Pituitary adenomas are almost always benign and their *spread* is only by local expansion. This leads to pressure on surrounding structures and creates the characteristic *clinical picture,* summarized as follows:

1. Pressure on the surrounding pituitary tissue, leading to hypopituitarism (amenorrhea or sterility, loss of libido, impotence, gradual loss of hair, and easy fatigue), the full syndrome of pituitary cachexia is rarely demonstrated.
2. Pressure on the sella turcica, leading to its ballooning and conspicuous enlargement.
3. Pressure on the optic chiasma, leading to visual field disturbances (bitemporal hemianopia, Fig. 15-4; or homonymous hemianopia).
4. Pressure on the posterior pituitary and the hypothalamus, causing diabetes insipidus.
5. Pressure on the third ventricle, causing signs and symptoms of increased intracranial pressure.

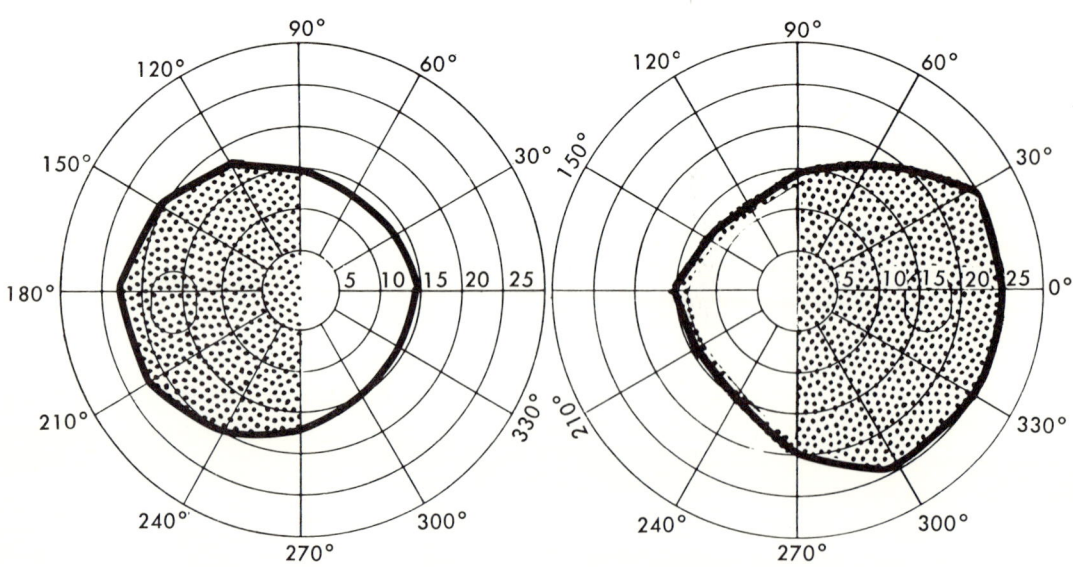

Fig. 15-4. Bitemporal hemianopia.

Pressure effects are more noticeable in chromophobe adenoma because they may reach a large size. If the tumor cells are functional (eosinophil and basophil adenoma), symptoms caused by excess hormonal effect ensue. Eosinophil adenoma causes acromegaly when it occurs in adult age groups, or gigantism when it occurs in younger age groups. Basophil adenoma causes Cushing's syndrome (see glossary).

Investigations necessary for diagnosis include skull x-ray films, angiograms, and pneumoencepholagrams, in addition to a very careful neurological examination (visual-field plotting and detailed fundus examination). Full hormonal assay including serum growth hormone and cortisol is important for assessment of the endocrinological state of the patient.

Treatment

Both radiotherapy and surgery are effective, but surgery is especially indicated in the presence of the following conditions: (1) Increased intracranial tension. (2) Rapid progression of visual deficits. (3) Pronounced endocrinological imbalance (severe hypopituitarism or excessive growth hormone). Extirpation of the tumor may be effected through a frontal craniotomy or transphenoidal approach.

Radiotherapy is indicated when none of the above conditions exist or when the patient refuses or is unfit for surgery. The last is not uncommon especially in patients suffering from pituitary deficiency.

Postoperative radiotherapy is indicated where surgery is not complete and is claimed to have diminished the incidence of recurrence (after surgery alone) quite substantially.

Technique of radiation varies. It may be either by external irradiation or interstitial implant.

For *external irradiation* highly penetrating sharply demarcated beams (6 Mev. supervoltage beam) are necessary. Multiple-field plan is also indicated to enable the delivery of a high dose to the tumor with a minimal dose to surrounding structures (especially the hyopthalamus and midbrain). The dose aimed at is usually 4500 to 5000 rads in about 5 weeks.

Interstitial irradiation is effected through a transphenoidal approach where 2 or 3 rods of ^{90}Y are implanted. The dose delivered is usually much higher than that by external irradiation, but the possible complications (cerebrospinal fluid leak with rhinorrhea, infection, and optic nerve and chiasma damage) are also more pronounced.

Prognosis depends on the extent of the tumor, neurological deficit at presentation, endocrinological balance, and possibility of full extirpation of the tumor. In chromophobe adenoma a combination of surgery and postoperative radiotherapy seems to afford the best results although radiotherapy alone yields a satisfactory outcome in a majority of cases.

CHAPTER 16

TUMORS OF BONE AND CARTILAGE

Bone tumors are of particular importance despite their rarity (3 per 100,000 population during adolescence) because they affect the young (generally below 20 years of age). They also occur in older age groups but mainly as a complication of a preexisting condition, such as Paget's bone disease. The fact that they are highly malignant (the 5-year cure rate is less than 20%) adds to their notoriety. The drama of the disease is sharply heightened by the radical nature of the treatment recommended, usually amputation or disarticulation of a limb.

A list of these tumors is shown in Table 16-1, but our discussion is limited to the types where radiotherapy plays a significant role. These types are osteosarcoma, Ewing's sarcoma, reticulum cell sarcoma, and metastatic bone disease.

BONE TUMORS
Osteogenic sarcoma (osteosarcoma)

Osteogenic sarcoma is the most common of primary malignant bone tumors and forms about one fifth of the whole group. It usually affects young subjects in the second decade of life with a 2:1 preponderance in males. It may occur in later years as a complication of Paget's disease of bone. Trauma had been claimed to be a *predisposing factor,* but no accepted statistical proof supports this premise. Chronic osteomyelitis, hyperparathyroidism, and exposure to ionizing radiation have been claimed to be other *predisposing factors,* with the latter being incriminated most strongly. The disease usually affects the metaphyses of the long bones, most commonly around the knee joint, but it may involve the epiphysis on rare occasions. The joint space itself and the lining cartilage are generally respected. The tumor leads to a dual process of bone destruction (mainly the medullary portion) and new bone formation attributable to periosteal activity (causing an onion-skin layered appearance, sunburst configuration, or Codman's triangle), leading to the characteristic radiological picture of osteogenic sarcoma. The tumor may *spread* beyond the confines of the bone to form a soft tissue mass. Osteosarcoma is characterized by early hematogenous spread with widely distributed me-

TABLE 16-1. Tumors of bone and cartilage

Tissues	Benign	Malignant
Primary		
1. Cartilaginous tissue	Chondroma Benign epiphyseal chondroblastoma	Chondrosarcoma
2. Osteogenic tissue	Osteoma	Osteogenic sarcoma (osteosarcoma)
3. Giant cell	Giant cell tumor	Giant cell sarcoma
4. Vascular tissue	Hemangioma	Hemangiosarcoma
5. Bone marrow		Ewing's sarcoma Multiple myeloma Reticulum cell sarcoma
6. Fibrous tissue	Fibroma	Fibrosarcoma
Secondary		
Cells from distant lesions (malignancies of breast, bronchus, etc.)		Metastatic bone disease

tastasis to the lungs, liver, and other splanchnic organs.

Among the important *complications* are local pathological fractures, severe general constitutional disturbances (fever, weight loss), and symptoms caused by metastases (such as hemoptysis if the lung is involved).

Investigations should include an x-ray examination of the diseased bone as well as the chest and skeletal survey (to exclude metastatic deposits). Bone scanning may delineate the intramedullary extent of the disease as well as distant metastatic deposits. Biopsy is an accepted procedure, provided that it is followed soon by the definitive treatment. Liver scan to exclude metastatic deposits is usually indicated. Blood chemistry studies (alkaline phosphatase usually high; serum calcium also high) and urine examinations (urinary calcium excretion high) are also indicated.

Treatment is usually surgical by amputation. Preoperative radiotherapy has been shown to be beneficial. A period of about 6 months of waiting after radiotherapy is recommended by some on the strength that most tumors that metastasize do so within this period. Such an occurrence would save the patient the severe psychological trauma of an unnecessary amputation. Recently a combination of surgery, radiotherapy, and multiple drug chemotherapy shows promise of improved results. *Radiotherapeutic technique* is applied by use of a cobalt-60 beam (uniform absorption of energy by bone and soft tissues). Fields employed are usually large and encompass the affected bone and adjoining joints, with an opposing parallel-field arrangement (Fig. 16-1). The dose aimed at is usually about 6500 to 7000 rads delivered in about 6 weeks.

The *results of treatment* are usually poor, the 5-year survival rate is within 20%. There are no recognized factors that are associated with improved prognosis. On the other hand, recent trials of combined approach may yield a better outcome.

Chondrosarcomas

Chondrosarcomas are the tumors next in frequency to osteogenic sarcomas among primary bone tumors. It usually complicates an already existing chondroma but it may arise anew. It appears more commonly in adult life (third to fifth decades). Ribs, pelvic bones, and vertebrae are the *bones most* commonly afflicted.

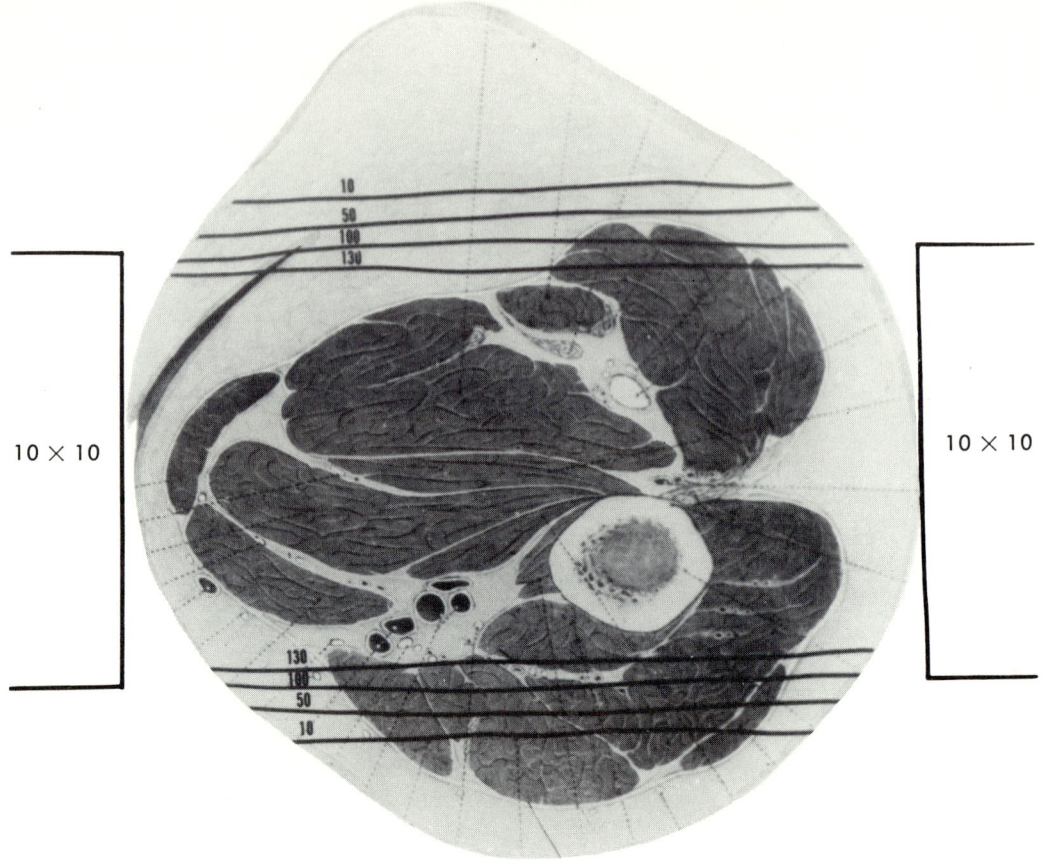

Fig. 16-1. Plan of treatment of a limb (thigh) by two opposing fields.

Lesions are slowly growing, and so the vascular supply remains relatively intact. Moreover its cells may be so well differentiated that sometimes it is difficult to differentiate it from a chondroma. Apart from local invasion, bloodborne metastases affecting the lungs are the commonest method of *spread*.

The *treatment* is largely surgical excision or amputation. Radiotherapy is recommended only when surgery is not feasible either because of the site of the disease (such as the vertebra), the extent of the disease (such as presence of bone metastases), or the general condition of the patient (poor surgical risk).

The technique and dosage of radiotherapy varies according to the goal of treatment; for example, pain relief would require less dosage than growth restraint. However, since the tumor is relatively radioresistant, generally high dosages are employed; for example, for growth restraint, a dosage of about 6500 rads is needed.

BONE MARROW TUMORS
Ewing's sarcoma

Ewing's sarcoma is a lesion of the bone marrow. The exact cell of origin is still disputable, but it is probably related to the reticuloendothelial tissue. The age incidence is somewhat earlier than in the case of osteogenic sarcoma.

As in osteogenic sarcoma the tumor *occurs* commonly in long bones, especially around the knee joint, but it may occur in pelvic bones. It leads to destruction of the bone associated with layers of periosteal new bone formation. This leads to the radiological picture of onion-skin appearance. Methods of *spread and pathological complications* are very similar to that of osteogenic sarcoma, with pain and general constitutional disturbances being the leading presenting symptoms.

This tumor is quite radiosensitive and can be controlled locally by radiotherapy. Nevertheless, its *prognosis* continues to be extremely poor (5-year survival rate about 10%), because of a high rate of distant metastases. The traditional method of *treatment* is radiotherapy, which may be followed by amputation in some cases. However, *recently the addition of intensive cyclical chemotherapy (actinomycin D, cyclophosphamide [Cytoxan], and vincristine) shows early promise of a significant increase in survivals*. The technique of radiation therapy is the same as that in osteogenic sarcoma.

Multiple myeloma

Multiple myeloma is a lesion that characteristically affects "multiple" sites. The cell of origin is considered to be the plasma cell. The tumor affects mainly the adults and elderly (75% of patients are in the fifth to seventh decades of life). There are three recognized *types* of myeloma: (1) solitary myeloma, which is usually a soft-tissue tumor occurring mainly in the upper air passages, (2) multiple myeloma, and (3) plasma cell leukemia. Some authors claim that the three types are linked and a patient who presents with a solitary myeloma may eventually develop the picture of multiple myeloma or plasma cell leukemia. Similarly a patient suffering from multiple myeloma may exhibit signs of plasma cell leukemia in the terminal stages of the disease.

Multiple myeloma usually affects flat bones (such as pelvic bones, vertebrae, ribs, and skull), but long bones also are often involved. The disease leads to widespread bone destruction, and splanchnic organs, such as the liver, spleen, and kidneys, are involved later. The peripheral and bone-marrow hematological picture may show a characteristic predominance of plasma cells. Serum proteins may be abnormal, with the appearance of special gamma globulins. The urine in some patients may contain abnormal proteins called Bence Jones proteins, which are pathognomonic of the disease.

Complications are usually from bone involvement (pathological fractures), or kidney involvement (renal failure), or hematological abnormalities (anemia). General debility, pneumonia, and various infections make a common picture of terminal illness.

Treatment to the generalized disease is usually by cytotoxic agents. Radiotherapy is indicated in solitary myeloma (treated radically and aiming at cure; a dose of 4500 rads is given in 4½ weeks) and where bony lesions cause symptoms (pain or impending pathological fracture). A dose of 3000 rads in 2 weeks is effective.

The *technique of radiotherapy* varies according to the site of the tumor treated. For a solitary myeloma in the region of the head and neck, a ^{60}Co or supervoltage beam is used. Fields should be of an adequate size, and a multiple field plan with proper protection to the surrounding structures may be used. The treatment of bony lesions is along the same lines for the treatment of bone metastases.

The *prognosis* of multiple myeloma is rather poor, with a 5-year survival rate of about 15%, whereas patients presenting with solitary myeloma stand the best chance for cure, with about one third of the patients living for 5 years.

Reticulum cell sarcoma of bone

Osseous reticulum cell sarcomas are relatively rare bone tumors that *originate* from reticuloendothelial cells of bone and may be confused histologically with Ewing's sarcoma. It affects both sexes equally during the second to fourth decades of life. Long bones are commonly affected, especially the tibia, femur, and humerus, but flat bones (such as the clavicle) may also be the site of origin.

This lesion is reputed to *spread* slowly, most commonly through a hematological route to other bones. When the disease extends to lymph nodes, one may have difficulty discerning it from a primary nodal reticulum cell sarcoma.

The presenting *clinical picture* is related to pathological fractures and pain. The lesion is sensitive to radiotherapy, and therefore this is the *treatment* of choice. The technique of radiotherapy is simple, with deployment of a ^{60}Co or supervoltage beam using two opposing fields to irradiate the whole bone and delivering a dose of about 4500 rads in about 4½ weeks.

Prognosis is relatively good, with a 5-year survival rate of about 35%.

Metastatic bone disease

Metastatic bone disease is the most common form of the bone malignancies. Bone metastases originate from carcinomas of the breast, prostate, lungs, kidney, thyroid, and stomach. Indeed, all primary malignancies that disseminate by the hematological route affect bone. Flat bones (vertebrae, pelvis, skull, ribs) are frequently involved, but long bones (femur, humerus) may also be affected.

Fractures are the most common *pathological complication,* but anemia caused by replacement of normal marrow and pressure on neighboring vital structures, such as the eye, from orbital metastases, and the spinal cord and nerve roots, from vertebral metastases, may occur.

The presenting *clinical picture* is invariably pain, which may be accompanied on occasions by neurological symptoms (such as paresis or paralysis). Rarely "silent" bone metastases are discovered as an incidental finding.

The *radiological appearance* is that of osteolytic lesions in most cases. However, lesions of prostatic origin are characteristically osteoblastic. The mixture of both osteolytic and osteoblastic pictures may be found on occasions.

Investigations other than x-ray and bone scans include biopsy, serum chemistry tests, and surveys of other systems when the bone lesion is the presenting clinical picture without a known primary.

Radiotherapy is the *treatment* of choice. It relieves the pain in most cases, but some lesions are known to respond rather slowly, such as those of prostatic origin. Radiation may help recalcification on certain occasions. However, irradiating a bone lesion in a long bone is not prophylactic against pathological fractures, and other measures including rest and artificial supports must be maintained.

The *technique of radiotherapy* is simple. The beam used depends on the site of the lesion. A metastasis in a superficially located bone (such as tibia, clavicle, and skull) may be treated easily with a conventional beam (250 kv.), whereas deeply located lesions (such as in the femoral neck) need a more penetrating beam (^{60}Co or supervoltage beam). The dose aimed at is about 3000 rads in 2 weeks or its biological equivalent.

As the treatment in these cases is necessarily palliative, *prognosis* regarding symptom relief is very good.

CHAPTER 17

MALIGNANT SOFT-TISSUE TUMORS

Under this chapter heading all malignant tumors of soft tissues other than those systems previously discussed are included. The different histological types are summarized in Table 17-1. Since all of these tumors are of mesothelial origin, malignant tumors are mostly sarcomas, largely highly malignant. These lesions are on the whole rare and form only 0.4% of all malignant tumors. Those of fibrous tissue origin are the commonest. Both *sexes* are almost equally affected and the *age incidence* is variable; for example, fibrosarcomas occur mostly in those who are below 50 years of age whereas rhabdomyosarcomas are more common in children and are known even in the newly born. Malignant soft-tissue tumors arise in *sites* related to their tissue of origin; for example, leiomyosarcomas are common in the gastrointestinal system where they originate from the plain muscles of the gut; liposarcoma originates in areas of fatty tissue such as in the buttocks or peritoneal fat; and fibrosarcoma originates in retroperitoneal fibrous tissues. However, since these tissues are found almost everywhere in the body, so can their tumors be found. Notwithstanding the site of origin or tumor bed, these tumors are capable of reaching large sizes, especially the liposarcoma and certain leiomyosarcomas. As a result, the tumor growth may outstrip its blood supply and such a condition leads to necrosis of its central part.

Histologically malignant soft-tissue tumors vary from the very well differentiated (as to make it sometimes difficult to distinguish from a benign tumor) to the extremely undifferentiated where one may not be able to define the tissue of origin. However, with the increasing familiarity and the introduction of electron microscopy many of these undifferentiated tumors are reclassified as rhabdomyosarcomas with the following different subgroups—embryonal (the most common), alveolar, and pleomorphic. The embryonal varieties occur chiefly in the head and neck region in children. Liposarcoma has two main subgroups—the myxomatous and the poorly differentiated.

On the whole the main method of *spread* is by local invasion. Lymph node metastases and spread by the bloodstream usually oc-

TABLE 17-1. Malignant soft-tissue tumors

Tissue of origin	Malignant tumors
Fibrous tissue	Fibrosarcoma
Myxoid or mesenchymal tissue	Myxosarcoma
	Mesenchymoma (mixed mesodermal tumors)
Fatty tissues	Liposarcoma
	Myxoliposarcoma
Smooth muscle (involuntary)	Leiomyosarcoma
Striated muscles (voluntary)	Rhabdomyosarcoma
Mesothelial tissue	Malignant mesothelioma
Synovial tissue	Synovial sarcomas
Vascular tissue	Kaposi's sarcoma
	Angiosarcoma
	Lymphangiosarcoma

cur late, except in the undifferentiated types or the embryonal rhabdomyosarcoma. Transcoelomic spread is particularly common in myxosarcoma.

The main *clinical picture* and pathological complications therefore are those of the local disease and its effect on surrounding structures. Disease occurring in the intraperitoneal or retroperitoneal tissues (such as fibrosarcomas) may lead to pressure symptoms, depending on the organ affected, such as intestinal obstruction (bowel), hydronephrosis (ureters), jaundice (bile ducts), pain (nerve roots or plexus), and edema or ascites (lymphatics). Should the tissue of origin be in the head and neck region, as with rhabdomyosarcomas, then pressure symptoms may produce a clinical picture of proptosis (eye displacement), nasal obstruction, sinusitis, or epistaxis.

Treatment of soft-tissue sarcomas is generally by wide excision. Sometimes this may take the form of amputation of an extremity or even more radical procedures, such as hemipelvectomy. On occasions, even this may not be feasible, depending on the tumor site and extent (peritoneal myxosarcomas or retroperitoneal fibrosarcomas). As a result of the aggressive spread of these tumors, local recurrence after surgery is common (90%), especially in the poorly differentiated tumors.

The role of radiation therapy is summarized as follows: As a first group, some soft-tissue sarcomas are quite radiosensitive and may be treated adequately with radiation alone. Such is Kaposi's sarcoma, which is a tumor of vascular tissue. This disease presents with a purple nodule (or nodules) in the extremities and moves in a "stocking-and-glove" fashion centripetally. There are often multiple subcutaneous deposits that are not appreciated by the clinician. The disease is controlled by a dose of 3000 rads in 3 weeks delivered to a large field.

A second group of tumors that are moderately radiosensitive are certain liposarcomas and fibrosarcomas, in addition to the embryonal rhabdomyosarcomas. A combination of surgery and radiotherapy is the best method of treatment because it ensures the longest survival and lowest recurrence rate. Wide excision of the lesion is followed by radiation as soon as the wound has healed. A dose of 6500 rads in 6½ weeks is recommended. Additional chemotherapy seems to improve the results of treatment in certain rhabdomyosarcomas.

The third group that is the most difficult to manage and carries the worst prognosis includes poorly differentiated fibrosarcomas and liposarcomas. A combination of radiotherapy and surgery is the method most recommended.

Technique of radiotherapy

The beam used is usually that of a cobalt unit or a supervoltage (4 to 6 Mev.) x-ray unit. *Field arrangements* depend on the site of the lesion, but they are usually kept simple, when possible, like a parallel opposing pair. However, complex techniques may be necessary, especially in the head and neck lesions. Large fields are usually the order of the day. Since a combination of large fields and high dose spells poor tissue tolerance, due care should be taken to protect adequately healthy surrounding structures. It is a good practice to avoid irradiating the entire width of an extremity in order to preserve a functioning limb.

Prognosis

Survival depends on various factors: histological type, grade of differentiation (high grade is half the survival of low grade), and site (the more peripheral the tumor, the better the results). Lesions distal to the knee or elbow are easier to control. The following outline shows the average survival-rate figures for the most common types:

Liposarcoma
  Whole group—30%
  Myxoid type—66%
Fibrosarcoma
  Well differentiated—70% to 80%
  Poorly differentiated—20% to 30%
Rhabdomyosarcoma—10% to 25%, but recent results seem to be substantially better, especially for limb tumors and for lesions that occur in children
Lymphangiosarcoma—Very poor

CHAPTER 18

CHILDHOOD MALIGNANT SOLID TUMORS

Table 18-1 lists tumors that occur early in life (first decade) with a peak in the first few years. Leukemia common in this age group is not included because it is not a solid tumor. The role of radiotherapy in its treatment is limited to the irradiation of the brain early in the management of the disease. Splenic irradiation or irradiation to local deposits (in lung, periosteum, and skin) may also be considered. Our discussion concentrates on the four most common types where radiotherapy plays an important role; they are medulloblastoma, neuroblastoma, retinoblastoma, and Wilms' tumor. Rhabdomyosarcoma and Ewing's sarcoma were discussed earlier.

The childhood tumors share the following characteristics:

1. Although these tumors are *not congenital* in the proper sense of the word, some may be related to chromosomal abnormalities (such as retinoblastoma).
2. All these tumors spread widely relatively early. Hematological spread to lungs, liver, bone, and brain are relatively common.
3. Some of these tumors may grow to reach large size and may present with general constitutional symptoms (fever, anemia).
4. Most of these tumors are noticeably radiosensitive.
5. The best line of management often is a combination of surgery, radiotherapy and chemotherapy.
6. Although 5-year survival rates are used in expressing the prognosis of these tumors as in other tumors, the results in a follow-up period equal to the child's age plus 9 months are usually significant.

MEDULLOBLASTOMA

Medulloblastoma forms about 6% of intracranial tumors and about 30% of childhood central nervous system tumors. Its peak incidence is between the ages of 2 and 7 years, but it may occur later in life. Both sexes are affected equally.

They originate from the residual cells of the external granular layer of cerebellum. The tumors arise frequently in the posterior midline or cerebellar vermis. From their

TABLE 18-1. Common childhood malignant solid tumors

Nervous tissue	
Central	Medulloblastoma
	Retinoblastoma
	Gliomas
	Ependymomas
	Craniopharyngiomas
Symphathetic	Neuroblastoma
Renal tissue	Nephroblastoma (Wilms' tumor)
Bone tissue	Ewing's sarcoma
	Osteosarcoma
Soft-tissue sarcomas	Rhabdomyosarcomas
Teratomas and embryonic sarcomas	
Liver	Hepatoma
Gonadal tumors	Granulosa cell tumor
	Dysgerminoma
Lymphoid tissue	Malignant lymphomas

site of origin they *spread* to affect the cerebellar hemispheres and fourth ventricle, resulting in interference with the flow of cerebrospinal fluid creating the clinical picture of increased intracranial pressure. These tumors have a predilection to spread to the spinal cord and cerebral hemispheres seeding throughout the subarachnoid space. Involvement of the cranial nerves and spinal nerve roots are the main *pathological complications* besides those attributable to increased intracranial pressure. The *clinical picture* depends on the extent of disease. However, symptoms and signs of increased intracranial tension (headache, vomiting, dizziness, and choking of optic disks) appear early. Disturbance of gait, loss of balance and coordination, muscle weakness, and nystagmus are common findings. Root pains or specific cranial nerve involvement usually occur late.

Investigations are performed along the same lines suggested earlier for intracranial tumors.

Treatment

Craniotomy and removal (by suction) of as much of the tumor as possible serves the dual function of histological diagnosis and relief of intracranial pressure. Sometimes it may be important to establish a shunt to relieve the pressure. Since the tumors are highly sensitive to radiotherapy, a postoperative course of external irradiation is the rule. Treatment volume includes both the whole brain and the spinal cord. The dose aimed at is about 3500 in about 4½ weeks to this whole volume with a booster dose of 1000 rads (in 1½ weeks) to the primary tumor site.

The most important complication of radiotherapy is bone marrow depression, which is noticeable during irradiation of the spinal column. The white cell count is a very sensitive indicator and invariably the treatment has to be interrupted if the count falls below 2000 per cm.[3] Isolation and special nursing care may be necessary in such cases. Other measures were discussed on p. 66. Other complications and their management are the same as in the treatment of gliomas (discussed earlier).

The *prognosis* is generally poor, with the 5-year survival rate being about 40%. The same factors that affect the general prognosis of tumors of the central nervous system (see p. 143) apply here.

NEUROBLASTOMA

Neuroblastoma is relatively rare (6% to 19% of childhood malignancies). It arises from any site containing elements of the sympathetic nervous system, but 40% of the lesions occur in the adrenal medulla. Most tumors develop in children under 4 years of age. Other common sites are the head and neck region followed by the thorax (especially the posterior mediastinum) and abdomen.

The lesion *spreads* widely by local extension as well as by lymphatic and blood-borne metastases early in its natural history. Abdominal and thoracic lesions show a stronger tendency for widespread metastasis than those tumors situated in the head and neck region. Bones (especially the long bones and skull), brain, and liver are among the sites most commonly affected, but no organ is immune.

The *clinical picture* depends on the site of origin as well as the extent of the lesion. Generally head and neck tumors present with a mass. Intrathoracic lesions present with pressure symptoms on mediastinal structures (esophagus with dysphagia, nerves with pain, vessels with edema, trachea with cough).

Apart from the usual *investigations*, the estimate of urinary catecholamines, dopamines, and vanillylmandelic acid (VMA) (metabolites of epinephrine and norepinephrine) may give an indication about the presence of a lesion or a recurrence after treatment and its extent. However, this is so only in lesions that secrete these hormones. Flat films of the abdomen or chest may show the tumor (calcification seen in plain films). Intravenous pyelography may help detect adrenal medulla tumors.

Complete excision is the best line of *treatment*. This is followed by postoperative radiotherapy if surgery was not complete, especially in intrathoracic and intraabdominal lesions. The fact that there are well-documented cases where the lesion showed signs of spontaneous regression (or maturation to the much less aggressive ganglioneuroma) should not dissuade one from active treatment because these incidents are unfortunately rare and unpredictable. The main *complications of radiotherapy* are marrow depression and retardation or stunting of growth of the irradiated vertebrae, causing scoliosis. Metastatic neuroblastoma has responded to combination chemotherapy.

Prognosis depends on the following factors: the age of the child (most favorable is below 1 year of age), the site of the lesion (head and neck is most favorable), the extent of the lesion (lack of lymph-node metastasis is favorable), and the degree of differentiation (the more differentiated are the more favorable). About 35% of all children treated are curable.

RETINOBLASTOMA

A retinoblastoma is a rare lesion arising from the reticuloblasts (nerve cells of the retina). It has a strong familial tendency (6% of all cases) and occurs in both eyes in about 30% of the patients. The peak age incidence is below 3 years of age. The tumor spreads locally to involve the whole retina, the optic disk, and optic nerve and eventually migrates into the meningeal spaces.

The main *clinical picture* is that of failing eyesight, a cat's eye reflex (whitened pupil by the underlying tumor) or secondary glaucoma. Examination of the eye by ophthalmoscopic examination reveals the retinal lesion. Other symptoms may stem from meningeal involvement (pain, neurological deficits).

Examination of the opposite eye is among the most important *investigations* to be carried out because it may reveal an early lesion that can be cured so that the child's eyesight is saved. Examination of other members of the family is also important. An x-ray examination of the orbital contents may reveal calcification on occasions.

Treatment depends on the extent of the lesion and the condition of the other eye. The most effective treatment is surgical excision. However, radiotherapy is indicated in the following conditions:
1. Lesion affecting the remaining eye. If the lesion is affecting about half of the retina, it may be possible to save the eyesight.
2. Postoperative radiotherapy (after enucleation of the eye) if the optic nerve is involved.
3. If the lesion involves less than one fourth of the retina, it is possible to cure it with radiation and to save the eye even when this is the only lesion.
4. If the lesion has extended to the meninges.

Surgery is usually carried by enucleation of the eyeball. Exenteration of the whole orbital contents is rarely indicated in advanced lesions. Postoperative radiotherapy is indicated when the disease has spread beyond the globe (paired wedge field to a dose of 4500 in 4½ weeks).

The *technique of radiotherapy* varies, depending on the objective of treatment and extent of disease.

Radiation to a small retinal lesion with preservation of the eye is carried out by sewing small cobalt disks (diameters of 5, 7.5, 10, and 15 mm.) to the retinal involved area and leaving it for about 7 days so that a dose of about 4000 rads is delivered. If the lesion is larger than a fourth of the retina, external irradiation may be applied (with preservation of the eyeball) by use of sharp beams (linear accelerator) and beam-directing devices to a dose of 3500 rads per 4 weeks.

The most important *complication of radiotherapy* is the disturbance of growth of the areas irradiated with an external beam (orbit and adjacent area of skull), leading to a certain degree of facial asymmetry. Eye complications such as iritis, panophthalmitis and retinovascular occlusions may occur with high doses.

Prognosis depends on the extent of the lesion and whether the disease is bilateral. As far as survival is concerned, the prospects are generally good, with failures in about 20% of patients treated. As far as saving the eyesight is concerned, successes are perhaps less frequent. In about half the patients, vision continues to be good. The other patients are left with varying degrees of visual deficits.

NEPHROBLASTOMA (WILMS' TUMOR)

Wilms' tumor forms about 12% of all malignant solid tumors in childhood. The average *age of incidence* is 3 years, but few cases are reported in the adult. They occur with equal frequency in both sexes.

Nephroblastoma arises from remnant mesodermal cells in the kidney. They *spread* by local expansion surrounded by a capsule, but eventually this capsule is broken, with extension of disease to the kidney tissue and perirenal structures. Sometimes the lesion reaches very large dimensions, occupying practically the whole abdomen. Widespread bloodborne metastasis (lungs, brain, liver) occur relatively early. Lymph node metastases are also fairly common.

The usual *clinical picture* is that of an abdominal swelling but abdominal and loin pains, low-grade fever, and anemia are other presenting symptoms.

Intravenous pyelography is the most important *investigation,* and findings are often pathognomonic. Chest x-ray, full blood count, and bone marrow examinations are other important tests.

The *treatment* that yields the best results is a combination of surgery (nephrectomy) and postoperative radiotherapy and chemotherapy. Postoperative radiotherapy is not recommended when the child is less than 1 year of age if the tumor is limited to the kidney and removed without spillage. Preoperative radiotherapy is indicated if the tumor is so large that it makes the tumor inoperable. Radiation reduces the tumor mass, making it resectable.

Prognosis depends on several factors: child's age (a younger child stands a better chance), presenting symptoms (fever and general constitutional disturbances are unfavorable signs), and the extent of the disease. The average 2-year survival rate is about 40%. However, better results (about 80%) have been reported more recently as a result of more active treatment with a combination of chemotherapy (actinomycin D) and radiotherapy. Indeed, even in the presence of distant metastases, an aggressive therapeutic approach is warranted.

CHAPTER 19

SKIN

Basal and squamous cell carcinomas of the skin are the commonest of all malignancies and are curable in the majority of cases. Generally, skin lesions grow slowly and are often discovered in early stages of development. The peak age incidence occurs during the seventh through the ninth decades of life. Generally, males who are fair skinned and work outdoors are the most susceptible individuals. The aging process (such as senile keratosis) and constant irritants, whether chemical or mechanical, are other *predisposing factors*. Such factors are particularly damaging to unhealthy skin such as burn scars, eczematous dermatitis, and so forth. Since a wide variety of treatment modalities, such as surgery, radiotherapy, chemical desiccation, and electric cautery, are employed, the indication for proper selection may depend on such things as the resultant cosmetic effect, the site of the lesion, and the time and cost to the patient.

Malignant skin tumors are summarized in the outline below. Our discussion concentrates on the three most important varieties; basal cell carcinoma, squamous cell carcinoma, and malignant melanoma.

Primary malignant tumors of the skin
    Primary tumors
        Epidermis
            Basal cell carcinoma
            Squamous cell carcinoma
            Malignant melanoma
            Paget's disease
        Dermis
            Vessels
                Blood vessels—hemangiosarcoma
                Lymph vessels—lymphangiosarcoma
                Kaposi's sarcoma
                Dermatofibrosarcoma
            Fibrous tissue—fibrosarcoma
            Nerve tissue—neurofibrosarcoma
            Muscle—leiomyosarcoma
            Lymphatic tissues—malignant lymphoma
        Appendages
            Sweat gland—adenocarcinoma
            Sebaceous gland—carcinoma
    Metastatic tumors
        From almost any primary, particularly from malignancy of the breast, lungs, and kidneys, and from non-Hodgkin lymphomas

BASAL CELL CARCINOMA (RODENT ULCER)

Basal cell carcinoma is by far the most common malignant tumor of the skin. It occurs more frequently in those exposed to excessive sun rays and outdoor conditions. Blonds and fair-skinned people are more susceptible. As both these conditions are very common in Australia, the disease is prevalent among the white outdoor workers, such as farmers. The lesion is commonly located on the hands and face (above a line drawn from the ear tragus to the angle of the mouth). It starts as a small papule that soon umbilicates and assumes the characteristic ulcer with its rolled everted edges. The only method of spread is by local invasion of the surrounding and deeper tissues, including bone, cartilage, or nearby vital structures (such as the eye). Lymph node or distant metastasis are almost unknown. Apart from *complications* resulting from local spread, some tumors may display foci of squamous cell carcinoma, which are on the whole much more aggressive.

Treatment of basal cell carcinoma is most commonly by surgery or radiotherapy. Surgery is especially indicated when the lesion has arisen in damaged skin or has invaded cartilage or bone. However, extensive lesions are often only curable by a combination of surgery and radiotherapy. The latter may be applied both preoperatively to diminish the size of the lesion and the extent of subsequent surgery, and postoperatively to margins where the disease is not fully excised. Radiation therapy is highly effective especially for lesions around the eye, ear, and nose, and when applied properly, cosmetic results are highly satisfactory.

The *technique* consists of single fields and relatively superficial beams (such as 100 kv.). The dose varies according to the size of the treated volume; for example, 4000 rads are given in 2 weeks to a 3 cm. circle and 5400 rads are given in 3 weeks to a 5 cm. circle. A 1 cm. rim of normal tissue must be included in the treatment volume, since small clones of tumor cells may be found adjacent to the clinical tumor. Lesions over bone and cartilage require a high quality beam and protracted fractionation. The reaction in the treated area may proceed to the stage of moist desquamation, but this heals in about 3 weeks, and healthy skin remains, except in the case of an extensive lesion, which may leave a superficial scar.

The *prognosis* of cure is excellent. Less than 5% of cases recur, usually at the edges of the lesion treated.

SQUAMOUS CELL CARCINOMA

The *predisposing factors* are similar to those of he basal cell carcinomas, summarized as follows:

1. Excessive sunlight and wind (as in countries near the equator), especially to the exposed parts of the body, such as the hands and face
2. Chemical carcinogens, such as tar or arsenic that may be ingested in some medications
3. Chronic irritation, such as pipe smoking, especially with the old-style clay ones
4. Precancerous skin condition, such as radiation dermatitis, eczematous dermatitis and senile keratosis

Clinically the lesion is usually an ulcerating one.

It *spreads* by local extension as well as lymph node metastases, which occur in about 7% of cases depending on the site of the lesion and the abundance of lymphatics.

Treatment depends primarily on the extent of the disease. The primary lesion may be treated either by adequate excision or radiotherapy. Radiotherapy is usually applied with a beam of moderate pentration (such as 200 kv.) through a single field. The dose given is usually about 6500 rads in 6 weeks. The treatment of metastatic lymph nodes may be a radical dissection if these are mobile and accessible. If the nodes are fixed and limited to one group, radiation therapy can sterilize them. The beam to employ then is generally a more penetrating beam (such as cobalt 60), and a multiple field plan may be necessary. A radical dose of about 6500 rads is usually given.

The *prognosis* is generally very good, with a cure rate of about 85% of the primary lesion. The picture changes quite appreciably if the lymph nodes are involved and may be grave if these are fixed or multiple.

Special sites

Squamous cell carcinoma of the vulva or the penis is essentially a skin lesion modified by the site of the primary tumor and by the relatively high incidence of lymph node metastases. Vulval lesions are more serious because the primary lesion may be extensive and bilateral. Lymph node metastases usually occur early and are bilateral. The best results reported so far follow radical vulvectomy and bilateral node dissection. However, early vulval lesions can be controlled by local radiotherapy with a radium or tantalum wire implant. An external beam can be used satisfactorily with a small volume and protracted fractionation. Lesions of the penis are treated successfully by radiotherapy, especially if they are limited to the skin without deep involvement. These have been discussed in more detail elsewhere. Other areas such as the dorsum of the hands and feet have a limited radiation tolerance because of the underlying tendon sheaths and are easier treated by surgery.

MALIGNANT MELANOMA

Malignant melanoma is the most serious skin disease. Its gravity is demonstrated by the fact that the 5-year crude survival rate free of disease in a series of about 500 patients reported by McLeod and his colleagues was less than 50%. Malignant melanoma represents just over 1% of all skin cancers. It is more common in people with fair complexions. It reaches a peak incidence around the age of 50 with females being the predominant sex. Melanoma of the vulva is an exception, since it occurs most commonly in those over 60 years of age.

It is claimed that there is an endocrine factor in the development of malignant melanoma, but no conclusive proof has been found to support any of the many theories advanced. A flat, hairless mole, pigmented light or dark brown, is a usual preliminary lesion to a frank malignant melanoma. A darkening in color, ulceration or bleeding of such a lesion, or rapid growth may indicate a malignant change (a hairy, elevated papillary mole rarely changes to malignant melanoma).

The lesion usually originates in the pigmented cells, melanocytes, which are mainly located in the deep layers of the epidermis. It is commonly found in the soles of the feet and in the head and neck region. Close to one half of the lesions arise from benign junctional nevi. Malignant melanoma *spreads* mainly by the bloodstream and lymphatics. A small primary lesion that may go unnoticed with widespread metastases is not unknown, and about one sixth of the patients suffer from metastases at presentation. The frequency of lymph node metastases varies according to the site of origin of the primary lesion. Those in the limbs have the highest incidence, with the axillary and inguinal nodes being the ones most commonly affected. Skin nodules are a common manifestation of spread along the lymphatic channels. Bloodborne metastases disseminate most commonly to the lungs followed by the liver, but any organ in the body may be affected.

Clinically these lesions are staged by the International Union Against Cancer (UICC) as follows:

T1 Lesion less than 2 cm. in diameter and less less than 1 cm. in depth
T2 Lesion 2 to 4 cm. in diameter and 1 to 2 cm. in depth without invasion of deep structures
T3 Lesion greater than 5 cm. in diameter, and invasion greater than 2 cm. in depth; satellite nodules within 5 cm. of the primary

The nodal classification is along lines discussed earlier (see p. 84).

Investigations should include chest x-ray films, liver function studies (including a liver scan), and a bone survey. An excisional biopsy of the lesion with a wide margin (2.5 cm. on all sides) usually clinches the diagnosis.

Treatment of malignant melanoma is rather controversial. The most accepted policy consists of wide surgical excision of the local disease followed by dissection of the draining lymph nodes "en bloc." The role of radiotherapy is still not widely accepted in North America despite the good results reported by several authors (Ellis, 1946; Todd, 1946; Helleriegel, 1963; Sandeman, 1966; and Edwards, 1968). Wide excision of the primary lesion followed by radiotherapy to the draining lymph nodes is recommended for T1 cases, (Helleriegel, Ellis). Where there is clinical nodal involvement preoperative radiotherapy to the lymph nodes followed by complete surgical excision is claimed to lead to an improvement of the 5-year survival rate by a factor of about 50% (Sandeman, 1966).

The *technique* of radiation therapy is usually simple, in that a ^{60}Co or a supervoltage x-ray beam is used. Most of the draining lymph node areas are treated adequately by two parallel opposing fields. The dose aimed at varies from 5000 to 6000 rads in 5 to 6 weeks depending on whether the treatment is preoperative or definitive. A relatively new technique is endolymphatic injection of radioactive material. Radioactive gold (^{138}Au) or iodine is injected in the lymphatics draining the region of the primary lesion. The radioactive material is taken up and concentrated by the draining nodes, which are destroyed by the irradiation. However, this method has not met with wide acceptance as it is rather complicated and the concentration of the radioactive materials by the nodes is not regular and sometimes insufficient, especially when the node is heavily involved with malignant disease.

Prognosis depends on several factors among which are as follows:
1. Clinical stage of the disease. The 5-year survival rate for T1 and T2 is about 70% and 45%, respectively.
2. Sex. Females on the whole do better than males.
3. Age. Younger patients do better than older ones.
4. Extent of the primary lesion. Patients with a superficially infiltrating lesion are known to do better than those with deeply infiltrating ones.

BENIGN SKIN DISEASES

Benign skin diseases are rarely treated by radiotherapy because of the possible late sequelae of radiation (malignant transformation, genetic damage). There are, however, certain skin disorders that find their way to radiation departments when other therapeutic modalities fail to relieve the clinical problem at hand. Radiation if properly delivered can contribtue to palliation or cure. Not all disorders so treated will be covered, nor will the chronic dermatitides be included in this discussion for these latter diseases are for the most part treated by dermatologists.

Keloid is treated only when it is recurrent or symptomatic (itchy, red, and tender or painful). In the first case a single dose of radiation (300 to 600 rads) is given, followed by excision and a further dose of radiation, within 24 hours after operation. Such a line of management is claimed to reduce both recurrence and bulkiness of the lesion. Postoperative radiotherapy alone (600 to 1200 rads) may achieve the same result. In case of a symptomatic lesion, the treatment is usually expectant and the dose varies according to response. It should be kept to as minimal as possible with strict limitation of the treatment volume to the edges of the keloid. With recent advances in plastic surgery the necessity of treating keloids with radiation is fortunately becoming rare.

Plantar warts occur mainly in young adults and are believed to be caused by a virus. Resistance to the usual treatment of surgical paring followed by salicylic acid application can result in a somewhat disabled painful foot. Radiotherapy delivering 400 rads every third day for a total of 1200 rads is generally successful. A superficial beam (75 kv.) is used and repeated treatment for recurrence is to be avoided.

GLOSSARY

abscopal effect a measurable response of tumor tissue definitely separate from the area treated; found in chronic leukemias or in lymphomas where irradiation of an enlarged spleen or lymph nodes cause a generalized disease remission in the former and relief of obstructive symptoms in the latter.

absorbed dose a measure of the amount of energy absorbed from a radiation beam, by a medium in the path of the beam, described in units of rads. One rad is equivalent to 100 ergs of energy deposited per gram of absorbing material.

absorbed dose rate the rate of deposition of energy in an absorbing medium. It is measured in units of rads per unit time.

absorption of radiation any material placed in the path of a radiation beam will absorb some of the radiation, that is, some of the energy of that beam. The amount of absorption will depend upon the type of radiation, the density of the absorbing material, and the atomic number of the absorbing material. This may result in ionization, heating, production of scattered radiation, and rearrangement of atomic bonds.

acromegaly this condition is caused by an abnormally increased secretion of growth hormone after puberty resulting in generalized overgrowth of skeletal and soft tissues. Eosinophil adenoma of the anterior lobe of the pituitary may lead to such a disorder.

afterloading techniques in these techniques, hollow applicators (designed to carry a radioactive material) are implanted or inserted into the volume to be treated. These are checked by various methods (x-ray films or image intensifier) before the radioactive material is inserted, a step that is usually done when the patient has been transferred back to his (or her) room. Its main advantage is that it allows the operation to be carried out without any exposure of personnel to radiation. It also limits the radiation exposure to specified personnel who are closely monitored. The most commonly used afterloading technique is that used in the treatment of carcinoma of the cervix (Fig. 1-15).

apposition plate a flat plate that may be put on the end of the front pointer, perpendicular to the central axis of the beam; used in skin apposition.

backpointer an attachment to a therapy treatment machine used in conjunction with a frontpointer or front light beam to align the direction of the radiation beam. It consists of a curved arm, arcing over the patient, with a pointer lying along the central axis, pointing to the exit point of the radiation beam.

backscatter some of the radiation after entering the tissue will scatter back toward the surface. This portion of the radiation is called backscatter. Therefore, the *surface* or *skin dose* may be defined as the *air dose* plus the *backscatter dose*

$$D_{skin} = D_{air} + D_{BS}$$

Backscatter depends on the following three factors: size of treatment field, depth of irradiated part, and quality of the x-ray beam.

1. *Field size (FS)*. Backscatter increases with increasing field size. A larger beam irradiates a larger volume of tissue, with a resultant increase in scattered radiation. This, in turn, produces more backscatter, adding to the surface exposure dose.
2. *Depth*. Only when the thickness of the irradiated part exceeds the range of the scattered radiation will full backscatter occur. Thus the amount of radiation scatter backward will increase to a maximum (depend-

ing on the energy of the radiation) as the thickness of the irradiated part increases, to a critical value. After this thickness is reached, a further increase in thickness will contribute no additional backscatter.

3. *Quality of x-ray beam.* As the radiation energy increases, the backscattter will increase until a maximum is reached. This occurs when the energy has a half-value layer of 1 mm. of copper. In beams with a higher HVL, scattering occurs more and more in a forward direction. Consequently, there is less backward scattering, and the backscatter decreases.

Backscatter is independent of treatment distance.

Example of backscatter:

With 250 kv. and with HVL = 1 mm. of copper, the surface dose can vary from a few percent to 49% (FS = 20 × 20 cm.^{2}) over the air dose. Whereas a cobalt-60 beam varies from a few percent to 6% (FS = 20 × 20 cm.^{2}).

This shows the importance of backscatter in orthovoltage therapy.

beta plaque a flat plate or curved surface that is coated with a radioactive material and emits electrons. It is placed on the surface of the area to be treated. The depth of penetration is very small, in the order of millimeters. A common isotope used is strontium 90. An example of a beta plaque is an ophthalmological applicator, curved to conform to the surface of the eye (Fig. 1-18).

betatron a machine that accelerates electrons to high energies by means of a varying magnetic field. These electrons can be used for patient treatment or can be directed toward a target to produce a beam of high energy x rays. The betatron installed at the Manitoba Cancer Foundation has a maximum energy of 35 Mev.

breast bridge a jig used to set up tangential fields, in particular, for treatment of the breast or a remaining skin flap.

bolus any material that may be placed on an irregular or sloping surface of a patient or a phantom to provide a flat surface perpendicular to the central ray of the radiation beam. Tissue-equivalent materials such as wax or rice are usually used. A bolus serves to even out the dose delivered to the target volume.

buildup a feature of high-energy or supervoltage photon beams, in which the maximum dose is not delivered to the surface of the patient, but at some depth beneath the surface. The absorbed dose "builds up" to its maximum, at a depth that increases with photon energy. For example, the depth of the maximum is 0.5 cm. for cobalt-60 radiation, and approximately 4 cm. for 30 Mev. x rays. This results in a skin-sparing effect.

cesium 137 this radioactive isotope is commonly used in the form of tubes and in teletherapy equipment. It has a half-life of approximately 30 years and emits a gamma ray of 0.66 Mev.

cesium-137 tubes used instead of radium for intracavitary insertions, especially in the treatment of carcinoma of the cervix. They are cylinders 2 cm. in length and approximately 4 mm. in diameter, usually calibrated as milligram equivalent of radium.

cesium teletherapy unit mainly used to treat head and neck tumors. A large source of cesium contained in a shielded housing provides a beam of useful radiation. The patient is normally situated at approximately 30 cm. from the source. This is a relatively short SSD unit (see p. 14).

cast a shell, usually of plastic, individually formed to fit the outer shape of the patient. All relevant external radiation field markings are placed on the case. During treatment, the cast holds the patient in one position and ensures that the tumor volume is treated exactly.

cobalt 60 an isotope useful in radiotherapy because of its relatively long half-life (5.27 years) and its high-energy gamma rays. Two gamma rays are emitted in equal numbers, one at 1.17 Mev. and the other at 1.33 Mev. It is commonly used in teletherapy equipment, but can also be used in the form of beads and needles for interstitial and intracavitary therapy.

cobalt-60 beads radioactive beads approximately 8 mm. in diameter used for intracavitary insertions to irradiate the endometrium. Since they can be packed in to fill the uterus, they produce isodose curves that follow the contours of the uterus, giving a more homogenous dose to the tumor volume than can be obtained with tandem sources.

cobalt-60 teletherapy equipment a treatment machine consisting of a large source of cobalt 60 (in the order of 3000 to 5000 curies) placed in a shielded housing with an opening protected by movable shutters. With these shutters in the open position, a useful beam of radiation emanates from the opening. This beam can further be defined by a set of diaphragms, which control the field size. The patient is placed at a large distance from the source, to improve the penetration of the beam (because of the inverse square law) and to decrease the penumbra. Standard source-to-skin distances are 60 to 100 cm.

collision loss (see *radiation loss*)

collimator a beam control mechanism included in the head of almost all radiotherapy units. Its function is to outline the limits of the beam and thus control the field size. It is usually constructed of heavy metal rods.

Compton (absorption) process Compton in 1923 predicted that an electron in collision would recoil from the point of interaction. Thus the incident energy or photon (causing the collision) is divided between the recoil electron and the scattered photon. Therefore the total absorption coefficient is divided into an absorbed portion and a scattered portion. In a collision of a low energy photon, the scattered photon has nearly the same energy as the primary photon, with only a small amount of energy given to the recoil electron. In a collision of a high-energy photon, the situation is reversed and the recoil electron acquires most of the energy of the primary photon.

cone a cone-shaped attachment to a radiation machine, through which the beam passes and which limits the cross-section to the desired size. A complete set for various field sizes are usually available for each machine.

contact therapy treatment by an x-ray machine designed for use at very small TSD (target-to-skin distance) of 1 to 5 cm., at relatively low energy (approximately 60 kv.). Useful for small skin lesions.

contour an outline of the patient taken in the plane of treatment on which all relative external skin markings are placed and within which the tumor volume is localized. This facilitates treatment planning.

conventional therapy treatment by x-ray beams, not in the supervoltage range.

Cushing's syndrome a clinical syndrome described by Cushing and caused by hypersecretion of the adrenal cortex from hyperplasia, adenoma, or carcinoma. Increased hormone secretion causes metabolic and sexual disorders, including obesity, fatigability and weakness, amenorrhea, impotence, hirsutism, edema, glycosuria, osteoporosis, cutaneous purple striae, and hypertension.

diaphragm the part of a radiation beam therapy machine that limits the field to the desired size. The thickness of the metal required increases with the energy of the beam. For units in which the diaphragms are the only field-limiting component, they will be adjustable to allow for various field sizes. Diaphragms may also be used in conjunction with cones to collimate the field.

dose distribution a map of the treatment volume and adjacent tissues that indicates the relative dose received by these tissues when one or more fields are used to treat the patient. The dose is indicated by means of isodose curves drawn on the contour of the patient. The following are various terms connected with "dose distribution":

D_0 *dose* dose needed to kill 67% of the cells in a tissue culture.

dose rate rate at which any given dose is produced by the treating unit; for example, it is about 80 rads per minute in most 250 kv. units. It depends on the target-to-skin distance (the shorter, the higher). In addition to this factor, it depends on the activity of the source in ^{60}Co units. In supervoltage units it may be as much as several hundred rads per minute.

dose time this expression is used to relate the dose delivered in a particular situation to the total number of days during which this dose was given.

erythema dose dose of radiation (usually a beam of 250 kv.) enough to produce skin erythema.

integral dose dose that represents the total energy absorbed from the beam by the patient. It was defined by Prof. Mayneord in 1942.

sublethal dose dose that is unable to kill the cell though injurious to it.

electron therapy treatment by electrons accelerated to high energies by a machine such as the betatron. Used mainly for lesions situated at or near the surface. The advantage is that unlike x rays, electrons deliver the maximum dose to the first few centimeters of tissue, with the depth increasing with increasing energy, and then the doses decrease relatively rapidly with increasing depth, thus sparing the tissues beneath.

endocrine gland glands in which no definite duct system exists. Secretions pass into the blood directly. An example is the pituitary gland.

entrance port the area on the surface of a patient or phantom on which a radiation beam is incident.

erg a unit of work or energy. The fundamental unit of work is the dyne centimeter. 1 dyne centimeter = 1 erg. Work is measured as the product of the force exerted and the distance through which the force acts.

exit dose the dose at the point where the axis of the beam emerges from the patient.

exit port the area on the surface of a patient or phantom through which the beam leaves the patient or phantom.

exocrine gland gland characterized by having external ducts or ducts through which their secretion is expelled. An example is the parotid gland.

exposure dose a measure of the quantity of radiation delivered to a point by a source of radiation, measured in units of roentgens, based on the ability of x or gamma radiation to produce ionization. A dose of one roentgen is delivered to a point if, because of the ionization of air at that point, one electrostatic unit of charge is produced per cubic centimeter of air at standard temperature and pressure.

field size the dimensions of the cross section of the radiation beam. It may be defined in a number of ways. For example, it is the width of the 50% isodose curve in air at the required SSD.

filter an insert, composed of various layers of different metals (aluminum, copper, lead) put in the x-ray beam to filter out the lower energy rays of the beam.

fixed-field setup treatment by one or more stationary fields orientated at various angles as opposed to a moving field setup.

focus-to-skin distance (FSD) The distance between the focus of an x-ray tube and the skin of a patient.

fractionation the technique whereby, rather than delivering one large dose of radiation to the tumor volume, a number of smaller doses are given at regular intervals for a prescribed length of time, such as 6000 rads in 6 weeks.

front pointer an attachment to the head of a treatment machine that points along the central axis of the beam. The tip of the pointer is at a distance from the source equal to the desired SSD.

gamma ray radiation emitted from a radioactive isotope. It is electromagnetic in nature and consists of photons of one or more discrete energies.

genes the molecular complexes that control the morphology, development, and behavior of an organism.

gigantism abnormal secretion of growth hormone in the prepubertal period causing increased growth of the body or enlargement of a part (such as the hands and feet). Often used synonymously with acromegaly (in the adult). Results from eosinophil adenoma of the anterior lobe of the pituitary gland.

gold 198 a radioactive isotope used in interstitial therapy in the form of seeds, 2 mm. long, or in intracavitary therapy in the form of a colloidal solution. The isotope has a half-life of 2.7 days and emits photons predominately at 0.41 Mev.

half-life period the time required for half the number of atoms of a radioactive isotope to disintegrate or decay. The decay of a radioactive source is represented in Fig. 1-15 where radon is studied. Table 1 shows the half-life period of the most commonly used isotopes.

half-value layer (thickness) (HVL) a measure of the quality of the radiation. Indicates the thickness of the specified material required to reduce the intensity of the radiation beam to one half of its initial value. For example the HVL of ^{60}Co is 11 mm. of lead.

Horner's syndrome a combination of clinical findings including contraction of the pupil (myosis), drooping of the eyelid (ptosis) and loss of sweating over one side of the face (anhydrosis). It results from paralysis of cervical sympathetic innervation.

hyperbaric oxygen treatment the radiation treatment is carried out while the patient is in a pressure tank (usually under 3 atmospheres of pressure) in an oxygen atmosphere, after having been

TABLE 1. Half-life periods of commonly used isotopes

Phosphorus	^{32}P	14.3	days
Cobalt	^{60}Co	5.2	days
Yttrium	^{90}Y	20	years
Iodine	^{131}I	8.05	days
Cesium	^{137}Cs	30	years
Tantalum	^{182}Ta	115	days
Gold	^{198}Au	2.69	days
Radium	^{226}Ra	1620	years
	(in 0.5 mm. of platinum)		

there for a time. The purpose is to oxygenate anoxic regions in the tumor and thus make them more susceptible to radiation damage.

image intensifier a device incorporated in recent diagnostic x-ray machines or simulators that is capable of intensifying the x-ray picture in such a way that it can be seen on a monitoring television screen. It enables the operator to examine any organ or check any radioactive implant with little exposure to radiation of personnel.

interstitial insertion a technique of radiation therapy whereby an array of sources in the form of needles, seeds, or wires is inserted into the tumor volume according to a set of rules called the Paterson-Parker system.

intracavitary insertion a technique of radiation therapy whereby an array of radiation sources is placed in a cavity so as to irradiate the surrounding tumor. Examples are radium or cesium tubes in the uterus and vagina; colloidal gold in the peritoneal cavity or pleural cavity.

inverse-square law a physical law describing the intensity of radiation at various distances from a point source. The intensity of radiation is inversely proportional to the square of the distance from a point source.

iodine 131 a radioactive isotope with a half-life of 8 days. Administered internally, it tends to concentrate in the thyroid. Used in the treatment of hyperthyroidism and thyroid cancer.

isodose curve a curve on which all points receive an equal radiation dose. A series of them will map out the relative intensities of a radiation field in a phantom or patient.

LD_{50} a term that represents a single total-body irradiation lethal in 30 days to 50% of a group of animals. For man it is about 350 to 450 rads.

lead shield sheets or slabs of lead of the appropriate thickness are shaped and inserted in the beam to protect sensitive regions.

LET (linear energy transfer) LET is usually expressed in kilo electron volts per micron and gives the rate at which energy is deposited along the track of the ionizing particle. Heavy particles of protons or neutrons produce denser tracks (and consequently a large LET) compared to electrons the tracks of which have a small LET (or less ion pairs). Generally, particles and dense tracks have a high RBE.

leukopenia reduction in the number of leukocytes or white blood corpuscles.

light beam most supervoltage therapy units are equipped with a light beam that simulates the direction and field size of the radiation beam, allowing us to visualize the area to be irradiated. Cross hairs usually indicate the central ray.

linear accelerator a high-energy x-ray machine that accelerates the electrons to their final energy by a series of electrostatic kicks from a linear ray of accelerating electrodes. The electrons then impinge on a target, to produce high-energy x rays.

localization films x-ray films taken with various radiopaque markers in order to localize the position of the tumor relative to the external markings.

mold the general class of treatment aids manufactured specifically for an individual. Specific items may include positioning casts, wax bolus, lead masks, and surface applicators.

moving-field setup treatment by a beam moving in a predetermined manner about the patient or treatment while the patient is moving in a predetermined manner about the radiation source. Two examples are a rotational treatment whereby the source moves in a continuous arc at a constant radius about the patient, and a pendulum setup whereby the source moves back and fourth to treat a relatively narrow tumor volume. The advantage of a rotational treatment is that the tumor dose is much greater than the skin dose.

multiple-port treatment to deliver a high dose to the tumor volume at a depth without destroying the tissue near the surface, one may direct more than one radiation beam toward the tumor from different angles in order to increase the dose to the tumor relative to the skin. Also called crossfire technique.

output refers to the dose rate that can be expected at a certain point from a particular radiation machine. When used in conjunction with the percentage depth dose to the tumor and the required tumor dose, the treatment time can be calculated.

oxygen-enhancement ratio for a given lethality, anoxic cells require two or three times the dose required for well-oxygenated cells. The ratio of the former dose to the latter is called the oxygen-enhancement ratio. This is demonstrated graphically in Fig. 7-1. Heavy particles have a low oxygen-enhancement ratio (OER).

penumbra the region at the edge of an irradiated volume that receives some radiation, but not the full dose of the beam. It exists because of the finite source size and from scattered radiation.

percentage depth dose the dose delivered to a point at a certain depth in a phantom divided by the maximum dose delivered to the phantom ($\times 100$). The maximum dose is at the surface of the phantom for conventional radiation and at a particular depth in a phantom for supervoltage radiation. The percentage depth dose will increase until the depth of the maximum and thereafter will decrease at a rate determined by the quality of the radiation.

phantom a mass of tissue-equivalent material used for dosimetry purposes. May be cubical in shape or specifically contoured to simulate the shape of a particular part of the body. Common materials are water, wax, Perspex, or a special rubber material (Fig. 3-4).

phosphorus 32 a radioactive isotope that emits beta rays and has a half-life of 14.3 days. It is administered internally, in solution, and tends to concentrate in the bone marrow, spleen, liver, and lymph nodes. Useful in treatment of polycythemia vera.

photoelectric (absorption) effect a photoelectron is created when an electron from the K shell of an atom is removed as a result of interaction with a quantum of energy. All the energy of this quantum is acquired by the resultant photoelectron. The atom becomes an excited (unstable) atom and after a short time another electron will fill the K shell to produce a characteristic radiation that is very soft.

photon refers to the discrete bundles of energy, or quanta, that are electromagnetic in nature and emitted by a radioactive material, or by an x-ray machine, such as gamma rays and x rays.

pin and arc an attachment for a therapy unit used to position the beam at a specific angle and aimed toward a specific point in the patient.

Plummer-Vinson syndrome this syndrome consists of dysphagia associated with hypochromic anemia and occurs in women. There may be atrophy of the mucous membrane of the cricopharyngeal area in the esophagus. A good diet and iron seem to control this abnormality.

point A an imaginary point described by Todd and Meredith as being 2 cm. lateral to the cervical canal and 2 cm. above the cervical os. The point is supposed to lie in the paracervical tissues.

point B a reference point that lies 3 cm. lateral to point A and is used as a means of evaluating pelvic wall dosage.

primary beam the direct radiation beam emanating from the head of the irradiating unit. Scattered radiations result when this beam collides with any object (patient, treatment table, walls).

quality the penetrating power of a photon beam, described in terms of half-value layer.

radiation loss when a high-speed electron collides with a target atom, the two following types of losses occur: (1) Collision loss from the collision between the high-speed electron and the orbital electrons of the target atom. The product of this collision is mainly heat. This happens when the high-speed electron is of low velocity or the target material is of low atomic number, such as water. (2) Radiation loss from collision (or very close approach) between the high-speed electron and the nucleus of the atom. The electron will lose almost all of its energy, and radiation (or a photon) is produced. This radiation is called *bremsstrahlung*, which is a German term that means 'braking radiation' because the nucleus of the target stops or brakes the high-speed electron.

radium a radioactive isotope commonly used for radiotherapy. It has historical importance in that it was the first isotope to be used medically and is used as a radiation standard. The half-life is about 1620 years and photons of many discrete energies are emitted up to a maximum of 2.2 Mev. It is used in the form of needles and tubes for interstitial and intracavitary insertions.

radon a radioactive isotope existing in the form of a gas. One of the decay products of radium 226. Its use is now obsolete because of the danger of using a gaseous radioactive material and because of the availability of other radioactive isotopes. The half-life is 3.83 days. It used to be sealed in glass capillary tubes and used in the same manner as gold seeds for permanent implants.

recoil electron an electron that has been set into motion by a collision or by a process involving the ejection of another particle or electron. The direction and magnitude of the recoil are determined by the conservation of momentum.

relative biological efficiency (RBE) dose of reference radiation to produce a given biological effect as related to a dose of test radiation to produce the same biological effect. It is used to compare the biological effect of a certain type of radiation to a reference type of radiation, usually of orthovoltage quality.

REM this unit is used in protection work to calculate the dose absorbed by personnel when exposed. It is the quantity of any ionizing radiation that has the same biological effectiveness as 1 rad of x rays.

Dose in rems = (Asborbed dose in rads) (RBE_p)

where RBE_p is the relative biological efficiency of the offending radiation.

scatter when a material is in the path of a radiation beam, the material not only absorbs some of the radiation, it also scatters some in all directions, usually reducing the quality of the beam at the same time. Therefore the radiation received at a point has two components: scattered and primary. It follows that the exposure rate at a point in air will be increased if a patient or phantom is placed behind it. This is caused by "backscattered" radiation.

simulation films x-ray films taken with the same field size, source-to-skin distance, and orientation as a therapy beam in order to mimic the beam and for visualization of the treated volume on an x-ray film.

skin apposition a method of setting up a treatment beam whereby the beam is angled until the end of the cone or the end of an apposition plate is flush with the surface of the patient in the region of treatment.

skin sparing because of the buildup of the absorbed dose in supervoltage radiation deep to the skin, the skin surface does not receive the maximum dose delivered. The skin reaction is therefore much less than would be expected from conventional radiation.

source-to-skin distance (SSD) the distance from the source to the skin of the patient.

split course a course of radiotherapy delivered in two parts separated by a period of rest varying from 2 to 3 weeks.

sublethal less but usually only slightly less than lethal.

superficial therapy treatment with an x-ray machine of relatively low energy, approximately 100 kv. Penetration is not large.

supervoltage therapy treatment with gamma radiation or x-radiation of over 1 Mev. energy.

suprapubic cystotomy an operation aimed at opening the bladder through a suprapubic skin incision.

whole-body irradiation a technique whereby the whole body is irradiated to a low uniform dose in a specially designed installation. The exposure dose rate can be made approximately uniform in a volume $9 \times 9 \times 6$ feet high by strategic placement of a number of sources around this volume.

thrombocytopenia reduction in the number of thrombocytes or platelets. Megakaryocytes, which give rise to platelets, are the least radiosensitive of the myeloid elements but are still damaged by moderate doses of radiation. They are slow to recover from radiation damage in comparison to the rest of the myeloid series.

INDEX

A

Abbe, Robert, 2
Abscopal effect, 66, 162
Absorbed dose, 162
Absorbed dose rate, 162
Absorbed portion, 164
Absorption coefficient, 164
Achalasia, 100
Acidophil adenoma, 139
Acoustic neurinoma, 139
Acromegaly, 162, 165
Actinomycin D, 149, 157
Adenoid cystic carcinomas, 87, 103
Adrenalectomy, 111
Afterloading techniques, 162
Air dose, 162
Alcoholism, 100
Alkaline phosphatase, 109, 147
Alpha particles, 17
Alveolar ducts, 68, 151
Alveoli, 85, 96
Alveolus, 89
Amenorrhea, 144
American Radium Society, 3
Anal canal, 85
Anal carcinoma, 103
Anaphase, 51, 52
Anaplastic tumors, 82, 87
Anderson, C. D., 3
Angiosarcoma, 152
Anhydrosis, 165
Aniline dyes, 130
Ankylosing spondylitis, 67
Anorexia, 96
Anterior commissure, 92
Antibody, 66
Antidiuretic hormone, 96
Antigen-antibody, 66
Antral tumors, 89
Antrectomy, 90
Apposition plate, 162
Aqueduct, 141
Aromatic amines, 130

Arrhenoblastoma, 121
Arsenic, 81, 159
Aryepiglottic folds, 92, 93
Arytenoids, 92, 93
Asbestos, 81, 96
Ascites, 121
Astrocytes, 140
Astrocytomas, 139, 140, 143
Ataxic phase, 60
Atomic bonds, 162
Atomic number, 162
Atrium, 68
Axilla, 108
Axillary nodes, 109
Axon, 61

B

Back pain, 131
Backpointer, 46, 162
Backscatter, 36, 162, 163, 167
Bartholin's gland, 114
Basal cell carcinoma, 158
Basophil, 144
Basophil adenoma, 139, 145
BCNU, 136
Becquerel, 1
Benign skin diseases, 161
Benign tumors, 81, 82
Beryllium, 17
Beta particles, 17
Beta plaque, 163
Betatron, 3, 15, 163, 164
Bilharziasis, 130
Bladder, 41-42, 128-129
Bladder carcinomas, 130
Bleeding, 88
Block dissection, 99
Bolus, 44, 112, 163
Bone marrow, 135
Bone marrow transfusion, 72
Bone necrosis, 11
Bone pain, 88, 98
Bone tumors, 146

Bragg curve, 17
Brain edema, 143
Brain metastases, 98, 108
Brain scan, 143
Brainstem, 140
Braking radiation, 167
Breast, 107, 143
Breast bridge, 163
Bremsstrahlung, 167
Bronchioles, 68
Bronchogenic carcinoma, 143
Bronchoscopy, 96
Bronchus, 95, 96
Buccal mucosa, 98
Buildup, 13, 16, 163

C

Calcification, 83
Calcium, 71, 108
Caldwell Luc operation, 89
Californium, 17
Calyces, 128
Capsular distention, 88
Carcinogens, 81
Carcinoid syndrome, 96
Carina, 97
Carotid body tumor, 139
Cartilage, 95
Cast, 163
Cast forming machine, 30
Catecholamines, 156
Cat's eye reflex, 156
Celiac nodes, 87
Cell-mediated, 66
Cell survival curve, 75
Central nervous system, 139
Cerebellum, 61, 140, 141
Cerebral peduncles, 141
Cerebrospinal axis, 139
Cerebrospinal fluid, 141, 145
Cervical canal, 113
Cervical chain, 91, 98-99
Cervical esophagus, 100
Cervical lymphadenopathy, 92
Cervical nodes, 94, 101, 108
Cervix, 113, 114
Cesium (^{137}Cs), 7, 13, 163, 165
Cesium teletherapy unit, 163
Cesium-137 tubes, 163
Cesium units, 14
Cholesteatoma, 139
Chondroma, 147
Chondrosarcomas, 147
Chordoma, 139
Choriocarcinomas, 113, 121, 125
Chromophobe, 144
Chromophobe adenoma, 139, 144, 145
Chromosomes, 51, 54
Chronic anemia, 100
Chronic dermatitides, 161
Chronic glomerulonephritis, 68
Cigarette smoking, 96
Circumcision, 114
"Cleansing" simple mastectomy, 111

Clinical staging, 83
Clubbing, 96
Clubbing of finger, 69
Coal tars, 96
Cobalt (^{60}Co), 7, 13, 24, 163, 165
Cobalt disks, 157
Cobalt-60 beads, 163
Cobalt-60 teletherapy equipment, 163
Codman's triangle, 146
Coelomic spread, 82-83
Cold spot, 19
Collimator, 14, 163
Collision loss, 8, 163, 167
Colloid carcinomas, 107
Colloid cysts, 139
Colloidal gold, 24
Colonic tumors, 102
Colpostats, 117
Comedo carcinoma, 107-108
Compazine, 72
Compton, 11
Compton (absorption) process, 163
Compton scattering, 13
Cone, 61, 164
Congenital extropy, 130
Contact beam, 11
Contact therapy, 7, 25, 164
Continuous arc, 166
Contour, 164
Conventional therapy, 164
Conventional x-ray beams, 7, 11
Cooper's ligaments, 108
Cord, 92
Cord paralysis, 104
Coronal sulcus, 123
Corpus callosum, 141
Cortex, 61
Corticosteroids, 136
Cortisol, 145
Cranial fossa, 91
Cranial nerves, 91
Craniopharyngiomas, 139-140, 155
Craniotomy, 141
Curie, Madame, 3, 17
Curie, Marie and Pierre, 1
Cushing's syndrome, 96, 145, 164
Cutaneous anergy, 135
Cyclophosphamide, 136, 149
Cyclotron, 3, 17
Cylindroma, 103
Cystadenocarcinoma, 121
Cystitis, 131
Cytological studies, 88
Cytotoxic agents, 136

D

Decay, 13
Decay of radon, 22
Deep cervical nodes, 85, 103
Dehydration, 102
Delayed hypersensitivity, 135
Denture, 98
Depth dose, 35
Dermatofibrosarcoma, 158

Desquamation
  dry, 57, 111
  moist, 111
Deuteron beam, 16
Deuterons, 7, 15, 17
Diabetes insipidus, 144
Diaphragm, 164
Diarrhea, 118, 127, 129, 131
Diffuse histiocytic lymphoma, 137
Diffuse lymphocytic lymphoma, 137
Diffuse mixed lymphoma, 137
Diplopia, 91
DNA, 53, 54, 77
D_0 dose, 164
D_0 value, 64
Dose distribution, 164
Dose maximum, 38
Dose rate, 17, 36, 56, 164
Dose time, 38, 61, 164
Dose time factor, 56
Doubling dose, 54
Doubling time, 82
Duct carcinoma, 107-108
Dysgerminoma, 121-122, 155
Dysphagia, 87, 88, 97, 98, 102, 105, 112, 136
Dyspnea, 87-88, 92, 105
Dysuria, 127

E

Earache, 98
Ectopic gastric mucosa, 101
Eczematoid lesion, 108
Eczematous dermatitis, 159
Edema, 95
Electromagnetic wave, 12
Electron beam, 15
Electron microscopy, 151
Electron therapy, 164
Electrons, 7, 9, 12, 14, 163
Embryonal carcinoma, 124-126
Embryonal rhabdomyosarcoma, 151
"En bloc" dissection, 161
Endocarditis, 96
Endocrine gland, 164
Endolymphatic injection of radioactive material, 161
Endometrial carcinoma, 118-119
Endoscopic studies, 88
Energy, 10, 164
Entrance port, 164
Eosinophil, 144
Eosinophil adenoma, 145, 162
Ependymoma, 139, 155
Epiglottis, 92-93
Epilation, 143
Epileptic, 141
Epinephrine, 156
Epiphysis, 146
Epistaxis, 91, 152
Erg, 164
Ernst applicator, 117
Erythema, 111
Erythema dose, 164
Erythematous, 57

Erythrocyte, 63-64
Erythropoietic series, 63
Erythropoietin, 63
Esophageal dilation, 102
Esophagectomy, 102
Esophagitis, 136
Esophagus, 100
Estradiol, 107
Estrogen, 107
Ethmoid cells, 89
Ethmoidal tumors, 89-90
Ewing's sarcoma, 146-148, 154-155
Exenteration, 156
Exit beam, 13
Exit dose, 164
Exit port, 164
Exocrine, 85
Exocrine gland, 164
Exploratory operations, 88
Exposure dose, 164
Extended radical mastectomy, 110
Extrapulmonary manifestations, 96

F

Facial nerve, 103-104
Fallopian tubes, 113
Fallout, 70
False cords, 92
Faucial arches, 99
Faucial pillars, 98-99
Femoral nodes, 113
Fever, 135
Fibroma, 147
Fibrosarcoma, 129, 147, 151-153, 158
Field size, 164
Fifth nerve, 91
Filter, 9, 11, 36, 164
Filtration, 35
Fistula, 103, 118
Fixed-field setup, 165
Fletcher-Suit applicator, 117
Focus-to-skin distance (FSD), 165
Follicular adenocarcinoma, 104-105
Fourth ventricle, 141
Fractionated irradiation, 76
Fractionation, 17, 75, 165
Frenum, 123
Friederick, 3
Front pointer, 165
Frontal lobe, 141
Frontal sinuses, 89
Functional pain, 88
Fundus, 118

G

Gametes, 51
Gamma beams, 7
Gamma ray, 13, 165
Ganglioneuroma, 139, 156
Genes, 165
Genetic death, 53
Genetic effect, 54
Germ cell tumors, 121
"Germinal epithelium," 121

Gerota's capsule, 128
Giant cell sarcoma, 147
Giant cell tumor, 147
Gigantism, 145
Gingiva, 98
Given dose, 39
Glans, 123
Glaucoma, 156
Glial cells, 140
Glioblastoma multiforme, 140
Gliomas, 140, 155
Glomerular hyalinization, 68
Glossitis, 99
Glottic region of larynx, 92-95
Gold (^{198}Au), 161, 165
Gold grains, 22, 131
Golgi apparatus, 52
Gonadostromal tumors, 125
Granulocytes, 64
Granulopoietic series, 63
Granulosa cell tumor, 155
Growth hormone, 145, 162
Growth restraint, 88
Gynecomastia, 96, 125

H

Half-life period, 13, 23, 25, 165
Half-value layer, 9, 163, 165
Hemangioendothelioma, 139
Hemangioma, 147
Hemangiosarcoma, 139, 147, 158
Hematemesis, 87
Hematocele, 125
Hematologic spread, 82
Hepatoma, 155
Hematopoietic system, 72
Hematopoietic tissues, 62
Hematuria, 118, 128, 130
Hemilarynx, 92
Hemoptysis, 96-98
Hermaphroditism, 122
Heyman, 119
Hiatus hernia, 100
High speed electron, 167
Hiroshima, 67, 71
Histopathological studies, 88
Hoarseness, 92, 98, 100, 105
Hodgkin's disease, 87, 134, 137, 138
Hodgkin's lymphoma, 134-136
Homo sapiens, 70
Homogeneous absorption, 12-13
Homogeneous dose, 39
Hormonal ablation, 111
Homonymous hemianopsia, 144
Horner's syndrome, 104, 165
Hot spot, 19
Hyalinization, 83
Hydrocarbon, 81
Hydrocele, 125
Hydronephrosis, 115, 127
Hyperalimentation, 102
Hyperbaric oxygen chambers, 74
Hyperbaric oxygen treatment, 165
Hypercalcemia, 96

Hypernephroma, 128-129
Hyperparathyroidism, 146
Hypertrophic osteoarthropathy, 96
Hypopharynx, 100
Hypophyseal tumors, 139
Hypopituitarism, 144-145
Hypothalamus, 144-145

I

Iliac nodes, 124, 127
Image intensifier, 165
Immune mechanism, 72
Immune response, 108
Immunity, 66
Implants
  single plane, 18
  double plane, 18
  volume, 18
Impotence, 144
Inferior vena cavagram, 129
Inflammatory carcinoma, 108, 112
Inguinal nodes, 113, 114
Inhomogeneity, 44
Insulinoma, 83
Integral dose, 39, 164
Intensity, 10
Internal mammary nodes, 108
Interphase, 52
Interphase death, 53
Interstitial cell tumors, 125
Interstitial implant, 114, 131
Interstitial insertion, 165
Interstitial radiation, 7, 17
Intestinal obstruction, 88, 118
Intestine, 85, 143
Intracavity insertion, 115, 165
Intracavity radium, 7, 117
Inverse-square law, 165
Inverted-Y field, 136
Iodine (^{131}I), 25, 105, 161, 165
Ionization, 162
Ionization chambers, 39, 46-47
Iridium seeds, 114
Iritis, 157
Irritation, 95
Isodose curve, 34, 165
Isotopes, 13

J

Jacksonian attack, 141
Janeway, H. H., 3
Jaundice, 152
Joliot-Curie, F., 3
Jugulodigastric, 85, 98-99
Jugulodigastric nodal station, 91
Junctional nevi, 160

K

Kaposi's sarcoma, 152, 158
Keloid, 161
Kerst, D. W., 3
Kidney, 128, 143
"Kiss" ulcer, 92
Kraurosis, 113

L

Labium majus, 114
Labium minus, 114
Laryngeal nerve palsy, 102
Laryngeal palsy, 83
Laryngeal paralysis, 104
Laryngectomy, 94, 99
Laryngopharynx, 85
Larynx, 85, 92, 94-95
Late prophase, 52
Lawrence, E. O., 3
LD_{50}, 64, 71, 165
Lead shield, 165
Leiomyosarcoma, 129-130, 151-152, 158
LET (linear energy transfer), 165
Lethal dose, 74
Leukemogonic effects of radiation, 67
Leukocytes, 54
Leukopenia, 166
Leukoplakia, 92, 98, 113, 130
Lhermitte's syndrome, 61
Light beam, 166
Linear accelerator, 12, 166
Lingual mucous membrane, 100
Liposarcoma, 129, 151-153
Liver, 135
Lobular adenocarcinoma, 108
Localization films, 37, 166
Lower deep cervical nodes, 86
Lumpectomy, 109-110
Lung hilum, 96
Lung scan, 97
Lymphangiosarcoma, 152-153, 158
Lymphangitic spread, 108
Lymphatic spread, 82
Lymphatic vessels, 66
Lymphocyte depletion, 134
Lymphocyte predominance, 134
Lymphocytes, 65
Lymphoepithelial tumors, 99
Lymphoid tissue, 62
Lymphoma, 137
Lymphoreticular tissue, 134
Lymphosarcoma, 87, 134, 137
Lymphosarcoma of the stomach, 102

M

Macrophages, 65
Malignant ascites, 103
Malignant lymphomas, 155, 158
Malignant melanoma, 143, 158, 160
Malignant mesothelioma, 152
Malignant mixed tumor, 87
Malignant neuropathy, 83
Malignant teratoma, 121, 125
Mammography, 109
Manchester applicator, 117
Mantle-shaped field, 136
Maxillary antrum, 88, 89
Maximum tumor dose, 39
Mediastinal ducts, 87
Mediastinal nodes, 101
Mediastinal pleura, 101
Medulla, 141

Medullary carcinoma, 107-108
Medulloblastomas, 139-140, 154-155
Megakaryoblast, 63
Megakaryocytes, 63, 167
Meiosis, 51
Melanocytes, 160
Melanoma, 139
Melena, 87
Meningioma, 139
Menstruation, 113
Mesenchymoma, 152
Mesic x rays, 17
Mesothelial tumors, 151
Metamyelocyte, 63
Metaphase, 51-52
Metaphyses, 146
Metastatic bone disease, 150
Midbrain, 145
Middle deep cervical nodes, 86
Midpoint dose, 39
Minimum tumor dose, 39
Mitochondria, 52
Mitoses, 51, 53, 82
Mix D, 35
Mixed cellularity, 134
Mixed parotid tumor, 103
Modal dose, 38
Modified radical mastectomy, 110
Moist desquamation, 57
Mold, 166
Mold-forming machine, 30
Monochromatic radiation, 9
Monoenergetic beam, 9
Motor functions, 141
Mouth, floor of, 98
Moving-field setup, 166
Mucinous carcinoma, 108
Mucoepidermoid carcinomas, 103
Mucoepidermoid tumors, 87, 104
Mucositis, 58
Mucous gland, 96
Mucous membrane atrophy, 99
Multicentric, 98
Multinodular goiter, 104
Multiple myeloma, 147, 149
Multiple neurofibromatosis, 139
Multiple-port treatment, 166
Murine virus, 107
Mutations, 54
Myelocyte, 63
Myeloid series, 167
Myosis, 165
Myxomatous, 151
Myxosarcoma, 152
Myxoliposarcoma, 152

N

Nagasaki, 67, 71
Nakayama, 102
Nasal cavity, 89
Nasal obstruction, 91
Nasopharyngeal tumors, 91
Nasopharynx, 89
Negative pi-mesons, 7
Negative pi-meson beam, 17

Neoplasia, 81
Nephrectomy, 129
Nephroblastoma (Wilm's tumor), 157
Nephrotomogram, 129
Neuroblastoma, 139, 154-156
Neurocytoma, 139
Neurofibroma, 139
Neurofibrosarcoma, 158
Neurogenic sarcoma, 139
Neuron, 61
Neuropathies, 96, 108
Neutron, 7
Neutron beam, 17
Neutrophil, 63
Nickel, 96
Night sweats, 135
Nipple, 112
Nitrogen mustard, 136
Nodal stations, 85
Nodes, 89
Nodular histiocytic lymphoma, 137
Nodular lymphocytic lymphoma, 137
Nodular mixed lymphoma, 137
Nodular sclerosis, 134
Non-Hodgkin lymphomas, 134, 137
Norepinephrine, 156
Normoblast, 63
Nuclear membrane, 52
Nucleolus, 52
Nucleus, 52

O

Oat cell carcinoma, 97
Occipital lobe, 141
Oculomotor nerves, 91
Ohngren, 89
Olfactory neurons, 61
Oligodendroglioma, 139
Onion-skin appearance, 146, 149
Oophorectomy, 111
Optic chiasma, 144
Optic disk, 140
Optic nerve, 145
Oral cavity, 85, 98
Orange peel (*peau d'orange*), 108
Orbital floor, 89
Orchiectomy, 125
Oropharynx, 85, 99
Osteitis, 127
Osteogenic sarcoma, 147
Osteoma, 147
Osteomyelitis, 146
Osteosarcoma, 147, 155
Output, 166
Ovary, 113, 121
Ovoids, 119
Oxygen enhancement ratio (OER), 74, 166
Oxygen tension, 74

P

Paget's bone disease, 108, 146, 158
Pain, 88
Palatal fenestration, 91
Palate, 89, 98
Pancoast's tumor (pulmonary sulcus tumor), 96, 98
Pancreas, 59, 143
Panophthalmitis, 157
Pantograph, 32
Papillary adenocarcinoma, 104, 106
Papillary carcinoma, 108
Papilledema, 140
Para-aortic node, 87, 124, 130
Paraesophageal, 101
Parametria, 115
Paranasal sinuses, 85, 88
Paraplasmic granules, 52
Paraplegia, 102
Parasternal nodes, 108
Parathyroid, 85, 105
Paresis, 141
Parietal lobe, 141
Paris applicator, 117
Parotid, 59, 85, 103
Parotidectomy, 103
Particle beams, 7, 15
Paterson-Parker system, 165
Paterson and Parker, 18
Pathological fractures, 11, 83
Pelvis, 41, 128
Pendulum setup, 166
Penetrating power, 166
Penile corpora, 123
Penis, 123
Penumbra, 14, 166
Percentage depth dose, 11, 36, 166
Pericardium, 96, 101
Perikaryon, 61
Perineum, 114
Peritoneal seeding, 113
Perivesical tissues, 42
Permanent sources, 7
Perspex cast, 31, 105
Phantom, 33, 35, 166
Pharnygeal wall, 99, 100
Pharyngectomy, 99, 100
Pharyngolaryngectomy, 100
Pharynx, 85
Pheochromocytoma, 139
Phimosis, 123
Phosphorus 32, 25, 122
Photoelectric (absorption) effect, 11, 166
Photon, 164, 166
Photon beam, 166
Pia mater, 140
Pin and arc, 166
Pineal tumors, 139
Pins, 32
Piriform fossa, 100
Pituitary adenomas, 82, 144
Pituitary glands, 59
Pituitary tumors, 144
Placental tissue, 133
Plantar warts, 161
Plasma cell leukemia, 149
Platelets, 64
Pleomorphic, 151

Pleomorphic adenocarcinoma, 87, 103
Pleomorphic adenoma, 87, 103
Pleura, 96
Plexiform neuroma, 139
Plummer-Vinson syndrome, 98, 166
Pneumoencephalograms, 141
Poincaré, 1
"Point A", 117, 166
"Point B", 117, 166
Pons, 141
Positron, 3
Postcentral gyrus, 141
Postcricoid region, 93, 100
Posterior triangle nodes, 91
Preauricular, 85
Precentral gyrus, 141
Prepuce, 123
Pressure, 88
Primary beam, 36, 166
Primary photon, 164
Procarbazine, 136
Progesterone, 118
Promegakaryocyte, 63
Promyelocyte, 63
Pronormoblast, 63
Prophase, 51
Proptosis, 136, 152
Prostate gland, 123, 126, 130
Prostatic carcinoma, 126
Protons, 15
Pruritus, 135
Pseudohermaphroditism, 122
Ptosis, 165
Pulmonary fibrosis, 97, 112
Pyloric spasm, 59
Pyometra, 115

Q

Quality, 166

R

Rad, 3, 18, 39
RaD + E applicator, 25
Radiation absorption, 11, 162
Radiation dermatitis, 159
Radiation erythema, 1
Radiation-induced leukemia, 67
Radiation loss, 8, 163, 167
Radiation myelitis, 97
Radiation myelopathy, 61
Radiation nephritis, 67
Radiation pneumonitis, 68, 69, 97
Radiation sickness, 71, 118
Radiation therapy, 44
Radical mastectomy, 110
Radical vulvectomy, 160
Radioactive colloidal gold, 103
Radioactive gold, 122
Radioactive iodine, 104
Radioactive ores, 96
Radioactive phosphorus, 24
Radiosensitivity, 74, 75
Radithor, 3
Radium (^{226}Ra), 17, 24, 165, 167

Radium application, 115
Radium implant, 20, 98
Radium molds, 124
Radon, 167
Radon seed, 23
Rando phantom, 47
RBE, 64, 167
Recoil electron, 13, 164, 167
Rectum, 85, 103
Relative Biological Efficiency (RBE), 64, 167
REM, 70, 72, 167
Removable implants, 17
Removable insertion, 23
Repair, 75
Renal angiogram, 129
Renal cell carcinoma, 128
Renal cortex, 128
Ret, 39
Reticulocyte, 63
Reticuloendothelial tissue, 62
Reticulum cell sarcoma, 87, 134, 137-138, 146-147
    of bone, 149
Retina, 61
Retinoblastoma, 139, 154-156
"Retropharyngeal syndrome of Villaret," 91
Rhabdomyosarcoma, 130, 151-155
Rhinorrhea, 145
Rods, 61
Roentgen, 39
Rotational treatment, 166

S

Salivary gland tumors, 103
Sarcoma, 139
Scalene node biopsy, 96
Scatter, 35, 167
Scattered photon, 13, 164
Scattered portion, 164
Scattered radiation, 162
Schwannoma, 139
Scirrhous carcinoma, 108
Sebaceous gland carcinoma, 158
Sella turcica, 144
Seminoma, 122, 124-126
Senile keratitis, 113
Senile keratosis, 159
Sense of smell, 141
Sensory cortex, 142
Shielding effect, 16
    of bone, 12
Sigmoid colon, 118
Silicone, 81
Simple mastectomy, 110
Simulation films, 167
Simulators, 34
Skeletal survey, 109
Skin appendages, 57
Skin apposition, 167
Skin atrophy, 112
Skin dose, 39, 162
Skin sparing effect, 12-13, 163, 167
Smegma, 114
Soft palate, 99
Solder wire, 32

Solitary myeloma, 149
Somatic mutations, 54
Source-to-skin distance (SSD), 14, 35, 36, 167
Specific activity, 15
Spermatic cord, 125
Sphenoidal sinus, 89
Sphingomyelin, 62
Spinal accessory, 91
Spinal cord, 61, 95, 102, 136
Spindle, 51
Spleen, 66, 135
Splenectomy, 136
Split course, 97, 167
Squamous cell carcinoma, 87, 158-159
  of vulva, 160
SSD, *see* Source-to-skin distance
Stem cell, 63
Stenosis, 58
Stockholm applicator, 117
Stomach, 85, 102
Stomach carcinomas, 103
Stridor, 87, 92, 105
Strontium (^{90}Sr), 25, 70-71, 163
Strontium-90 applicator, 25
Subglottic region of larynx, 92-95
Sublethal damage, 75, 167
Sublethal dose, 164
Sublingual glands, 59, 85, 103
Submandibular glands, 59, 103
Submandibular nodes, 85-86, 89, 98, 103
Submaxillary nodes, 85
Submental nodes, 85, 86
Superficial beam, 11
Superficial therapy, 167
Superior mediastinal obstruction, 96, 104, 135
Superior vena cava, 97
Superior vena caval obstruction, 88, 98
Superior venacavography, 96
Superradical mastectomy, 109-110
Supervoltage, 7
Supervoltage therapy, 167
Supplementary radiotherapy, 90
Supraclavicular nodes, 86, 108
Supraglottic region of larynx, 92-95, 100
Suprapubic cystotomy, 167
Suprarenal glands, 59
Sweat gland adenocarcinoma, 158
Sympatheticoblastoma, 139
Synchrocyclotron, 17
Synovial sarcomas, 152
Systemic radiation, 7

T

Tandem, 117
Tantalum (^{182}Ta), 165
Tantalum wires, 20, 114, 131
Tar, 159
Target, 8
Target-to-skin distance (TSD), 164
Tarsorrhaphy, 91
Telangiectasia, 58, 112
Telangiectatic vessels, 57
Telephase, 51
Telophase, 52

Temporal hemianopia, 144
Temporal lobe, 141
Temporal lobe epilepsy, 141
Tenesmus, 127
Teratocarcinomas, 121
Terminal bronchi, 96
Terrestial radiation, 70
Testis, 123-124
Therapeutic ratio, 74
Thermoluminescent dosimeters (TLD), 46-47
Third ventricle, 141, 144
Thoracic ducts, 87
Thorium, 70
Thrombocytes, 63, 167
Thrombocytopenia, 167
Thrombophlebitis, 96
Thrombopoietic series, 63
Thymus, 104
Thyroid, 59, 85, 104
Thyroid carcinoma, 25
Thyroid gland, 60
Thyroidectomy, 105
Thyrotoxicosis, 25
Thyroxin, 104-106
Tissue maximum ratio, 45
Tissue tolerance, 74
Tongue, 98-99
  base, 99
  posterior third, 99
  tip, 98
Tonsils, 98-99
Tornberg classification, 107
Toxic goiter, 104
Trachea, 93
Tracheobronchial tree, 85, 96
Tracheostomy, 95
Transitional cell carcinoma, 128, 130
Transurethral resection (TUR), 127
Trophic corneal ulceration, 91
True vocal cords, 92
TSD (target-to-skin distance), 164
Tuberculous adenopathy, 104
Tumor dose, 38
Tumorectomy, 110
Tungsten target, 16
Tunica albuginea testis, 124

U

Upper deep cervical chain nodes, 85-86, 89, 98
Uranium, 70
Uremia, 115, 127
Ureteral, 115
Ureters, 128, 131
Urethra, 123, 128, 131
Urethritis, 124
Urothelium, 129
Uterovesical junction, 115
Uterus, 113, 118-119

V

Vagina, 113
Vaginal adhesions, 118
Vaginal bleeding, 115
Vaginal fornices, 115

Vallecula, 93
Van de Graaff generator, 12
Vanillylmandelic acid (VMA), 156
Ventricles, 92, 141, 144
Ventricular band, 93
Ventricular cavity, 93
Vesical diverticula, 129
Vesicles, 52
Vinblastine, 136
Vinča, 71
Vincristine, 149
Visual centers, 141
Visual deficits, 145
Visual field, 144
Volume irradiated, 56
von Roentgen, Wilhelm, 1

Vulva, 113-114
Vulvectomy, 114
Vulvitis, 113

W

Wedge, 37, 40
White matter, 61
Whole-body irradiation, 167
Wilms' tumor, 129, 154
Woody edema, 57

X

X-ray tube, 8

Y

Yttrium (^{90}Y), 24, 25, 145, 165
Y-12 plan, 71

N

```
616.992  R13                    91872

RAFLA-DEMETRIOUS

INTRODUCTION  TO  RADIOTHERAPY
```

College Misericordia Library
Dallas, Pennsylvania 18612